When Your Life Is Touched by Cancer

Advance Praise for *When Your Life Is T*

"Riter's book of valuable, compassionate advice focuses on making the cancer journey as good as it can be. His thoughtful communication strategies for patients, families, friends, and professionals are practical; his insights from various perspectives, vital. I recommend it highly for patient education centers and for public, health, and hospital libraries."

— Candace Ford Gray, executive director
PlaneTree Health Library

"…Reading Bob Riter's wonderful book triggers that vivid CancerLand moment before I headed down the hall for the first time to my designated turquoise barcalounger in the Chemo Suite. Why? Maybe because it reminds me how important it is that patients in a health crisis receive information that is clear and helpful, sensitively written, and practical in nature."

— Alysa Cummings, cancer survivor
Author of *Greetings from Cancerland*

"Riter's uniquely smart-but-folksy voice works well when tackling straightforward issues like blood donations or complex, existential issues like the nature of hope after cancer.…If you are looking for a gift to give people whose lives are touched by cancer, *When Your Life Is Touched by Cancer* is just what the doctor ordered."

— Dr. Wendy Harpham, MD, cancer survivor
Author of *When a Parent Has Cancer:
A Guide to Caring for Your Children*

> *This book is dedicated to*
> *the staff, volunteers, and clients of*
> *the Cancer Resource Center of the Finger Lakes.*

Ordering
Trade bookstores in the U.S. and Canada please contact
Publishers Group West
1700 Fourth Street, Berkeley CA 94710
Phone: (800) 788-3123   Fax: (800) 351-5073

For bulk orders please contact
Special Sales
Hunter House Inc., PO Box 2914, Alameda CA 94501-0914
Phone: (510) 899-5041   Fax: (510) 865-4295
E-mail: sales@hunterhouse.com

Individuals can order our books by calling **(800) 266-5592**
or from our website at **www.hunterhouse.com**

When Your Life Is Touched by Cancer

Practical Advice and Insights for Patients, Professionals and Those Who Care

Bob Riter

Hunter House
PUBLISHERS

Hunter House Inc., Publishers
PO Box 2914
Alameda CA 94501-0914

Library of Congress Cataloging-in-Publication Data
Riter, Robert N.
When your life is touched by cancer : practical advice and insights for patients, professionals, and those who care / Bob Riter.—First edition.
pages cm
Includes index.
ISBN 978-0-89793-679-8 (pbk.)—ISBN 978-0-89793-680-4 (ebook)
1. Cancer—Patients—Attitudes. 2. Cancer—Patients—Decision making.
3. Cancer—Psychological aspects. I. Title.
RC262.R58 2013
616.99'4—dc23   2013010336

Project Credits

Cover Design: Brian Dittmar Design
Illustrations: Brendan Heard
Book Production: John McKercher
Developmental Editor: Jude Berman
Copy Editor: Susan Lyn McCombs
Indexer: Candace Hyatt
Managing Editor: Alexandra Mummery
Publicity Coordinator: Martha Scarpati
Special Sales Manager: Judy Hardin

Rights Coordinator:
  Candace Groskreutz
Publisher's Assistant: Bronwyn Emery
Customer Service Manager:
  Christina Sverdrup
Order Fulfillment: Washul Lakdhon
Administrator: Theresa Nelson
IT Support: Peter Eichelberger
Publisher: Kiran S. Rana

Printed and bound by Sheridan Books, Ann Arbor, Michigan
Manufactured in the United States of America

9 8 7 6 5 4 3 2 1   First Edition   14 15 16 17 18

Contents

Important Note

The material in this book is intended to provide a review of information regarding coping with a cancer diagnosis and treatment. Every effort has been made to provide accurate and dependable information. The contents of this book have been compiled through professional research and in consultation with medical and mental-health professionals. However, health-care professionals have differing opinions, and advances in medical and scientific research are made very quickly, so some of the information may become outdated.

Therefore, the publisher, authors, and editors, as well as the professionals quoted in the book, cannot be held responsible for any error, omission, or dated material. The authors and publisher assume no responsibility for any outcome of applying the information in this book in a program of self-care or under the care of a licensed practitioner. If you have questions concerning the application of the information described in this book, consult a qualified health-care professional.

Foreword

When I was five my mother found a lump in her breast. She was ordered to the hospital by her physician for a biopsy. A few hours later her left breast was gone. She was left with severe lymphedema and a sense of shame about her body that stayed with her for the remaining 10 years of her life, when the disease returned to attack the other breast and her lungs. I remember her saying, "I'm not supposed to know, but I have cancer." She died at the age of 46.

That story has shaped my life, influenced career choices, sensitized me to the struggle of not only patients but also families as they cope with serious illness. Certainly medicine has changed since her death in 1954. Patients are now required to give permission for surgery, treatment modalities have become infinitely more sophisticated, and the important role of family and friends has been accepted. Many types of cancer have come to be viewed as chronic illness rather than terminal disease. Cancer is not viewed as if it were the plague, as Susan Sontag so aptly describes in her groundbreaking work, *Illness as Metaphor*. Yet the word cancer, when pronounced in a doctor's office, still brings with it a sense of shock, fear, and confusion.

I have followed Bob Riter's career with interest and admiration. I first got to know him when we both served on the Board of Directors of the Ithaca Cancer Network (ICaN), a volunteer organization that provided support to cancer patients. Bob was at that time on the staff of what was then the Ithaca Breast Cancer Alliance (IBCA). As he described the information and services IBCA offered to patients and their loved ones, we discussed how important it was to find a way to expand this care to people with all types of cancer. A few years later, the Board of IBCA decided to become the Cancer Resource Center of the Finger Lakes, of which Bob is now Executive Director. This decision has touched the lives of thousands of men, women, and children in our community.

The columns collected in this immensely useful book come out of both Bob's personal experience with cancer and his years of counseling patients and those who support them. There is a practical wisdom to the way Bob addresses the issues: how to talk to your doctor, make informed medical decisions, cope with post-treatment anxiety, be most helpful to someone recently diagnosed or undergoing treatment. The columns contain ideas for maximizing comfort, both physical and emotional. And they reflect some of the struggles and victories of living with this potentially life-threatening illness. The writing is characterized by empathy grounded in realism; there is no false reassurance, nor is there deep pessimism. Instead there is a gentle reminder of the value of every day of our lives, and a reminder to people with cancer that they are not alone.

— Nina Miller
Retired Executive Director
Hospicare & Palliative Care Services of Tompkins County

Acknowledgments

Thanks to Sue Riter, Sally Neely, Donna Heilweil, Kerry Quinn, Marguerite Sterling, Kat Lynch, Bev Johnson, Irene Kolberg, Nora Maloy, Sue Sandritter, and Francine Montemurro who routinely provided encouragement and feedback on drafts of my columns through the years.

Thanks to the *Ithaca Journal* and its editor, Bruce Estes, for taking a chance on a regular column about living with cancer. And thank you to the *Ithaca Journal* and Gannett for granting permission for those columns to be compiled into this book.

Thanks to Hunter House Publishers for bringing my work to a much larger audience, and to Jude Berman, Susan Lyn McCombs, and Alexandra Mummery for their thoughtful and perceptive editing.

Thanks to Andrea Kutsko Staffeld, Cindie Frost, and Nina Miller for contributing their support and talents to the creation of this book. Thanks to the Social Service League of Ithaca and to the Legacy Foundation of Tompkins County for making this book a community project.

Thanks to the oncology professionals at Cayuga Medical Center for treating their patients with kindness and skill, and for welcoming me into their family.

Thanks to the staff of the Cancer Resource Center of the Finger Lakes—Jyl Dowd, Sharon Kaplan, and Kerry Quinn—for sharing the joys and challenges of this work with me.

Thanks to the many volunteers of the Cancer Resource Center who give of their time and of their hearts.

And special thanks to Sandy Meek True whose initiative and positive energy made this book happen.

Introduction

I first noticed a small lump under my left nipple one summer night. I wasn't especially concerned until a few weeks later when I noticed bleeding from that nipple. My reaction was more surprise than worry. I had assumed a man's nipple was more or less ornamental without plumbing behind it.

I went to see my family doctor who sent me to a surgeon who did a biopsy. The report came back: *breast cancer*. I was 40 years old, in good health, had no family history of the disease, but there I was writing "mastectomy" on my calendar for August 30. It was all quite surreal.

Although breast cancer is rare in men, it's essentially the same disease as it is in women. One difference is that men almost always undergo a mastectomy. Of course, losing a breast does not have the same significance for a man as for a woman. On the flip side, men are more likely to go around shirtless. I'm usually the only single-nippled fellow in the pool.

Shortly after being diagnosed, I opened a fortune cookie and read a message that said, "You have yet to live the best years of your life." At the time, I wasn't sure if I was supposed to find that comforting or worrisome, but it's proven to be true.

For more than 12 years, I've worked at the Cancer Resource Center of the Finger Lakes. Most of our work involves helping people through a cancer diagnosis and treatment. We listen, provide support, and create a sense of community.

I routinely talk with patients, their loved ones, and the professionals involved in their care. I often see miscommunications because patients hesitate to ask questions, loved ones make incorrect assumptions about what the patient really wants, and health professionals misjudge the patient's level of understanding.

I also lead patient support groups and lecture to providers. I hear what patients wish their providers knew and what providers wish their patients knew.

My goal in writing this book is to help patients, their loved ones, and their health professionals communicate more effectively. Above all, I want to empower patients to understand that they are in control of their care.

Each chapter in the book first appeared as a newspaper column about cancer that I write for the *Ithaca Journal*. Most columns were suggested by a question posed by a patient or a patient's loved one. I realized that other people probably had the same questions, so I began the column to share my observations with a broader audience.

This book maintains the feel of a column with short, stand-alone chapters. This seems to work for people just diagnosed with cancer because they tend to have brief attention spans. Their minds are spinning in a thousand directions and they tend to browse rather than read a book cover to cover.

Some chapters are written from my personal experience as a cancer survivor, and others are written from my perspective as a professional in the cancer world. Many incorporate both perspectives.

People often ask how cancer changed me. I began to worry less about the future and began asking myself if I was happy and making a difference in my community.

What I enjoy most is connecting with people touched by cancer and helping them have sometimes difficult conversations with their loved ones, friends, and health professionals.

That's what this book is all about.

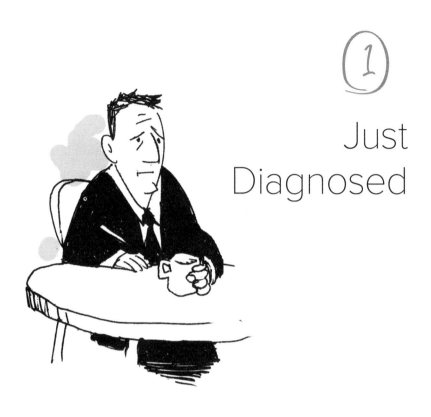

Just
Diagnosed

Advice for Those Newly Diagnosed

The first few days following a cancer diagnosis are like riding on top of a speeding train. You're hanging on for dear life and can't quite see what's ahead. Although every situation is somewhat different, this is what I generally suggest:

* Focus on one step at a time. If you are having a biopsy next week, focus on that biopsy and do not let your mind wander to what might happen next.

* Take someone with you to medical appointments. They can take notes and help you remember what was said.

✴ Do not hesitate to ask your doctor to repeat something.

✴ Be wary when family members, friends, and complete strangers say, "You should do…." Though well-intentioned, they do not know what is best for you.

✴ Know that you control whom you want to be told about your cancer diagnosis and when to tell them.

✴ Remember that cancer treatments change rapidly. What you hear from people who were treated in the past is out of date.

✴ Understand that cancer is not a single disease. What you hear about cancer in other people probably does not apply to your cancer.

✴ Remember that survival statistics are averages. They can be helpful if you want a general idea of the prognosis for people with your disease, but they can't predict what will happen to you as an individual.

✴ Do not hesitate to get a second opinion if you think it might be helpful. Your doctor won't mind. (If your doctor does mind, you should get another doctor.)

✴ Take a breath. A new cancer diagnosis is rarely a medical emergency. You generally have several days or even weeks to explore your options. (Some situations do require immediate attention—ask your doctor how long it is safe to wait before beginning treatment.)

✴ Do not begin a radical "cancer curing" diet or any major lifestyle changes before or during treatment. Just eat sensibly and nutritiously, exercise moderately, and get plenty of rest. You can make whatever lifestyle and diet changes you want after treatment is over.

* Conserve your energy for activities that are most important to you. Nearly everyone undergoing cancer treatment experiences fatigue. It is probably the most common and least publicized side effect.

* Do not be discouraged by the down days. Nothing goes in a straight line. You will feel better one day; then you will feel worse; then you will feel better.

Being diagnosed with cancer is life changing for many and life disruptive for nearly everyone. It is difficult at first, but once the decisions are made and treatment begins, most people gradually regain their rhythms. Cancer isn't fun, but treatment often ends up being more manageable than people expect. It's a club that no one wants to join, but trust me, you're in good company.

Good Cancers and Bad Cancers

I routinely talk with people who have just been diagnosed with cancer. They're struggling with treatment decisions and the realization that life is suddenly different.

I also talk with people with advanced cancer who are coming to terms with a poor prognosis and the realization that, in all likelihood, they will die prematurely because of that cancer.

It is particularly devastating to receive both rounds of bad news at once—that you have cancer and that a cure is unlikely.

In the regular world all cancer is bad, but in oncology offices there are good cancers and there are bad cancers. I realize that "good cancer" sounds like an oxymoron, but cancer professionals often think in those terms. Good cancers are generally curable.

Of course, if it's your cancer, it's never a "good cancer," a "garden variety cancer," or any other term that seemingly diminishes your fears or the disruption of your life.

Breast cancer and prostate cancer are the most common cancers (aside from skin cancer), and they're generally "good" cancers. People who receive these diagnoses undergo treatment and then return to their normal lives. In all likelihood, they will die many years later of something else.

But people who are diagnosed with the "bad" cancers often die from those cancers. New treatments are increasingly able to extend lives—often for many years—but a cure is the exception rather than the rule.

There are, however, survivors of even the worst diagnoses. I love meeting people who were treated for "bad" cancers years ago and are still going strong. There are no absolutes.

And many cancers fall somewhere in between being a good cancer and a bad cancer on the spectrum of cancer survivability. In some ways, people with these cancers have the most difficult time of all because statistics don't provide a clear roadmap for what's ahead.

Reality and hope aren't mutually exclusive. In fact, those of us who keep reality and hope in balance almost always seem to have an easier time—emotionally and physically—than those who lose that balance. Everyone with cancer has days of confidence and days of fear.

It's OK to Ask Your Doctor These Questions

People often leave their doctor's offices irritated with themselves for not asking what they wanted to ask. Sometimes they simply forget to ask. (I encourage people to bring a list). On other occasions, though, people aren't sure if it's OK to ask certain questions. Sometimes the questions that people hesitate to ask are the ones that they're most concerned about. These are some of those questions:

How much will this cost?

Being treated for cancer can be incredibly expensive. In general, you'll want to know what you'll have to pay out of your own pocket. Someone in the medical office should be able to give you a reasonable estimate of what your insurance will pay and what will be your responsibility.

Is there a less expensive alternative?

We all want the best possible care and physicians want us to have that care. But say, for example, that you have no health insurance at all and you're paying from your life savings. The newest and best drug for your cancer might cost $50,000 for a course of treatment. An older generation drug might be 95 percent as effective as the newest drug, but cost only $1,000. Is that a reasonable trade-off? It's an individual decision, but it's fair to ask the question.

What's the likely benefit from a proposed treatment?

Cancer treatment is about improving your odds of preventing a recurrence and extending your life. You can ask, "How much will this chemotherapy/radiation/surgery improve my odds of preventing a recurrence?" Sometimes the likely benefit is huge, sometimes the benefit is small, and sometimes it's uncertain.

Do I need ALL of the proposed treatments?

Sometimes the suggested treatment includes radiation AND chemotherapy AND hormonal treatment, etc. You can ask, "If I get chemotherapy, what's the added benefit of radiation? Or, if I get radiation therapy, what's the added benefit of chemotherapy?" We don't always have clear evidence, but these are reasonable questions to ask.

How long can I wait before beginning treatment?

Some cancers require that treatment begin quickly. Other cancers are slow moving and treatment can safely wait for many weeks. You can quite possibly spend time exploring other options or just going ahead with that long-planned vacation.

How long am I likely to live?

Some people want to know their prognosis and others don't. Doctor can't predict precisely how long you will live, but they can give you a general idea of what's typical for people with your condition. It's OK to ask. And it's OK not to ask.

Can you repeat that?

People usually miss a good deal of what their doctor tells them, especially if it's a stressful time. (Hearing that you have cancer is always stressful.) Don't be afraid to ask a doctor to repeat something.

Many of these questions don't have simple answers. People with cancer often have to make decisions with incomplete information. No one knows for certain how an individual will respond to a particular treatment or what the future might hold. Sometimes the answer to these questions will be, "I don't know" or "there's no data on that." But asking questions is always OK.

Second Opinions

People diagnosed with cancer sometimes ask me if their doctor will take offense if they get a second opinion.

The answer is no. Nearly all doctors today are receptive to patients getting second opinions. (And if you have one of those rare doctors who does take offense, you should seriously consider getting a new doctor.)

Your doctors want you to be comfortable with the treatment decisions that are made. And they want you to feel comfortable with them as individuals. Treating cancer is often a life-long partnership between the two of you.

Second opinions are especially beneficial when there are significantly different treatment options available. For example, surgery, radiation therapy, and "watchful waiting" are often reasonable options to consider for the treatment of prostate cancer. Talking with different types of physicians can be helpful, too.

Here are a few practical suggestions:

* It's entirely appropriate to ask your doctor for a recommendation as to where to go for a second opinion. This is especially true for rare cancers. You'll want a second

opinion from someone who sees that particular type of cancer on a regular basis. In addition, your doctor's office can help arrange the appointment and send a copy of your medical records for you.

* You should ask your doctor how long you can safely wait before beginning treatment. Some cancers are relatively slow moving and a month's delay in beginning treatment won't make any difference. Other cancers are more aggressive and treatment should begin quickly. It's sometimes reasonable to obtain a second opinion even after treatment has started.

* You should generally obtain the second opinion from a physician who is not associated with your first physician. Physicians who work together tend to share similar philosophies and practice patterns.

* You may be able to obtain a second opinion without leaving town by arranging a telephone consultation. Major cancer centers are often able to provide opinions based on your medical records.

* We usually think of second opinions in terms of treatment decisions, but it's also possible to request a second opinion on the pathology itself. That is, your slides can be sent to another institution for a different pathologist to review.

What should you do if your second opinion differs from the original recommendation? You can ask the two doctors to talk with each other to see if they can reach a consensus. You can seek a third opinion. Another option I recommend is to meet with your family doctor. He or she can often explain the options, place them in context, and help you reach a decision.

Cancer and Positive Thinking

Whenever someone is diagnosed with cancer, people feel compelled to say, "You gotta stay positive!" (This is usually said with an enthusiastic pump of the arm.)

I'm a pretty positive guy and I'm all in favor of positive thinking, but I cringe whenever I hear those words.

First of all, telling someone to be positive has never transformed anyone into actually being positive. I've yet to hear someone respond, "You're absolutely right. I've never thought about being positive, but now that you mention it, I see the wisdom in it. I will become positive and change my outlook on life." That just doesn't happen, at least not in my world.

My real concern is for people with cancer who may blame themselves for not being positive enough. How does one make sense of a recurrence if positive thinking is supposed to help? I hope no one sees their recurrence as the result of not thinking enough positive thoughts. People with cancer don't need another reason to beat themselves up.

Don't get me wrong—I think it's great to have a positive attitude when dealing with cancer. I did, and I'm sure it was helpful in my recovery.

If my cancer returns, I will again be positive. If there's only a 5 percent chance of survival, I figure that I'm going to be in that 5 percent.

But attitude is largely a function of personality, and you are who you are. Positive people enjoy having other positive people and positive energy around them. People who aren't so positive don't necessarily want or benefit from cheerleaders in the room.

And even the sunniest, most positive people will have down days when dealing with cancer. It's a scary, life-changing event, filled with uncertainty. Rather than telling them to be positive, acknowledge and share in their sadness on those days. Doing so can make for an honest connection.

Cancer is no different than every other aspect of life. We need to face it in our own way and on our own terms.

Surprising Facts About Cancer

I enjoy speaking with groups about cancer. I usually talk about my personal experiences and then describe cancer more generally and answer questions. After doing this for more than ten years, I know that certain facts always surprise people in the audience. Here are some of those surprises:

* If chemotherapy causes you to lose your hair, you'll likely lose all of your body hair—even the hair in your nostrils. That's why people on chemo sometimes have drippy noses. (The things we don't appreciate until there's a problem!)

* If cancer metastasizes, or spreads, from one organ into another, it doesn't become a second cancer. For example, if breast cancer spreads to a person's lungs, the cancer within the lungs is not lung cancer, it's breast cancer and is treated with breast cancer drugs.

✳ The lifetime risk for developing cancer in the United States is now one in three for women, and one in two for men.

✳ We often talk about cancer as being one disease, but there are more than 200 different types of cancer. They vary widely in terms of prognosis and impact on one's life. And our progress in treating each cancer varies as well— testicular cancer can now be cured even if it's relatively advanced. That's not true for most other cancers.

✳ Significant nausea from chemotherapy is now uncommon.

✳ Lung cancer kills many more women than breast cancer.

✳ The five-year survival mark is not magical. Some cancers can return ten or more years later. But the risk of a recurrence goes down for each year that passes cancer free.

✳ The end of treatment is often as psychologically stressful as the beginning of treatment. Making the transition back to "normal" is often unexpectedly difficult and slow.

✳ Fatigue is a nearly universal side effect of cancer treatment that people don't appreciate until it knocks them on their butts.

✳ Cancer is increasingly thought of as a chronic disease. We used to think that people were cured of cancer or they died. Now, people are often able to live with cancer for many years with a good quality of life.

✳ People often think of surgery, chemotherapy, and radiation as the three forms of cancer treatment. A fourth type of therapy—hormone therapy—can be just as important in the treatment of many types of breast, prostate, and other hormone-sensitive cancers.

✴ Chemotherapy and/or radiation are now sometimes given before surgery for certain types of cancer, including breast and rectal cancers. Shrinking the tumor may reduce the scope of surgery that's required.

Talking About Your Cancer

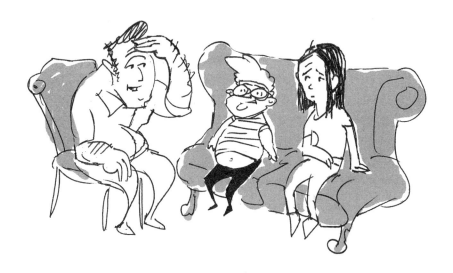

Telling the Kids

If you are diagnosed with cancer when you have young children, you're faced with what to share with them and how to share it.

It is important to realize that cancer affects the entire family and not just the person with cancer. As a member of that family, children have the right to be included.

Children can usually sense when something is wrong. And they will likely overhear the word "cancer" when you're talking with someone else. If you tell them the truth, they can focus on the reality rather than the even scarier things in their imagination.

When you talk with your children, it is important to use language they understand and to be sensitive to their concerns.

Here are a few suggestions:

* Children need to be assured of their own security. How will family life change as a result of what's happening? Who will pick them up from school? Who will make dinner? These questions come up even during a brief hospitalization.

* It's OK to say you don't know the answer to a question. This is often the reality with cancer—we may not know why something happened or what is going to happen next.

* You don't have to share everything at once. Several shorter conversations are often better than one long conversation.

* Encourage your kids to ask questions and set aside time for that purpose.

* Reassure them that cancer is not passed from one person to another. Nothing they did caused your cancer nor can they get cancer from you.

* Let them know about your treatment and any expected side effects. If you're going to lose your hair from chemotherapy, let them know in advance so they won't be surprised.

✳ Inform your children's school about your cancer so the teachers can be supportive and be alert for potential changes in your child's behavior.

✳ Be honest. Don't make promises that you may not be able to keep.

We all want these conversations to go perfectly, but don't be hard on yourself if you get tongue-tied or emotional. It's a hard time for everyone. Kids understand that, too.

Telling the Parents

I've seen many resources that provide advice on how to tell your children that you have cancer.

But what about the other generation—your parents?

Family relationships are sometimes complicated, so I don't presume to know what's best for you and your family, but some guidelines might be helpful.

In general, it's a good idea to talk openly with your parents about your cancer. Keeping secrets consumes energy when you could better use that energy for your own healing. And, if you don't tell your parents, someone else probably will.

But be prepared for your parents having a very emotional response to your cancer diagnosis, even if it's a cancer that's routinely curable. They will hear the word "cancer" and immediately assume the worst. Losing a child is a parent's worst fear.

Telling your parents might even uncover useful information about your family's medical history. A generation ago, there was a much greater stigma attached to cancer, so it wasn't often discussed, even within the family. Maybe they never told you that your grandmother and several aunts had breast cancer. This kind of information is important and should be shared with your physicians.

Problems sometimes arise with parents because they just want to help. This is especially true if they try to influence treatment decisions or otherwise exert control. You may need to gently remind them that you're the decision-maker on all matters relating to your illness.

This is one time in which it's absolutely OK for you to focus on what's best for you. If having your parents with you during cancer treatment is beneficial, then welcome them with open arms. If having them present is stressful, suggest other ways for them to contribute.

Tell them that they can always help by sending good thoughts and positive energy. But do try to keep them in the information loop. Everyone feels better when included.

"I have cancer. What's new with you?"

Two days after being diagnosed with cancer, I received a call from the Red Cross asking if I'd give blood in an upcoming blood drive.

I was a regular blood donor, so I received these calls a couple of times a year.

This time, my head nearly exploded with a thousand thoughts: Should I tell this anonymous person that I have cancer? Will she write, "Bob Riter has cancer" in some computerized database? Can people with cancer give blood?

I said, "Sorry, I can't make it this time."

When I hung up, I realized that I had been unable to say, "I can't give blood because I was just diagnosed with cancer."

The words "I have cancer" seemed to get stuck in my throat.

Nearly everyone who gets diagnosed with cancer struggles saying those words at first. It's an admission that you really do have cancer and that much in your life is suddenly so different.

The first people you tell are your family and close friends. That's emotional, but you know that they're somehow in this journey with you.

Telling more-casual acquaintances can be downright weird. People often ask, "How are you?" as a form of greeting. They expect to hear, "Fine. Yourself?"

A new cancer diagnosis makes "how are you?" a difficult question.

For weeks, I wrestled with what to say to whom. I'd ask myself, "How well do I know this person? Who are their friends and whom will they tell? Will their feelings be hurt if I don't tell them?"

No wonder shopping at the supermarket was exhausting. I had too many mental calculations to make when people asked, "Hi Bob. What's up with you?"

I once responded to a "how are you?" from a friend by saying, "Well, I was just diagnosed with breast cancer and I'm going to have a mastectomy next week and then a few months of chemotherapy. What's new with you?"

Although his expression was priceless, I decided that wasn't the smoothest approach.

As time passed, I became more relaxed about talking about my cancer. Nearly everyone was supportive, and many people stepped up and became dearer friends than ever before.

I did lose a few acquaintances. For whatever reason, they couldn't handle my having cancer and they gradually disappeared from my life. I think they weren't sure what to say at first and later felt awkward about never having said anything. (By the way, it's never too late to reconnect with those who have been ill. Small things like a card that says, "My thoughts continue to be with you" are always welcomed.)

It's now many years after my cancer diagnosis, and I'm about as open about my cancer as one can be. I'm not above showing my mastectomy scar to total strangers over dinner.

But I still remember how difficult it was for me to say, "I have cancer" when the Red Cross called that night.

My "Cancer Sucks" Button

I often wear a button that says cancer sucks. In addition to pretty well summing up the cancer experience, it's a great conversation starter.

Just last month, a man tapped my button as I was waiting in line for coffee in the San Antonio airport. He nodded sadly and told me that his young daughter was being treated for cancer in Houston. Since the button seemed to strike a chord with him, I asked if he'd like to have it. At first he shook his head, but I assured him that I had more in my office. He took it from me, attached it to his coat, and left to catch his flight.

It was one of those fleeting moments of shared humanity. We talked for only a few seconds, but the connection was real.

That's the thing about cancer. It allows us to connect with others by a kind of shorthand that cuts across the usual boundaries of gender, race, age, and class.

When I meet someone with cancer, or affected by cancer, I have a fairly good idea of what they're experiencing.

But it's important to realize that I don't know *exactly* what they're experiencing. Every cancer is different and every individual is different. This was brought home recently when a woman affected by a head and neck cancer told me, "I envy you people with breast cancer because you can put on your shirt and cover your scars."

That gave me pause.

Cancer can bring people together for another reason as well: It's a great equalizer.

An acquaintance was reading about a celebrity diagnosed with cancer and said she didn't have much sympathy for him because he had the money and connections to get the best possible care.

My reaction was quite different. When you're diagnosed with cancer, you're scared no matter how famous you are or how much money you have.

That's one of the reasons I wear my button. Cancer is scary, but it's a little less scary if we talk about it.

Don't Ask About My Battle

We struggle with language when the topic is cancer.

We don't think twice when cancer is discussed in military terms. When I was diagnosed with breast cancer, countless people told me to "fight this thing." Since I'm still alive, I'm often referred to as a survivor. If I were to die, my obituary might well read, "Bob lost his long and courageous battle with cancer."

The language of cancer seems to mirror the language of war. Battles are won and lost. There are survivors and there are victims. But is this the language we should be using?

Saying that someone lost his battle to cancer seems to blame him for not fighting hard enough.

I'm not quite comfortable being referred to as a survivor of cancer. Survivor is a better term than victim, but survivor seems to indicate victory. I'm not sure that I have beaten cancer. There's always the chance it might come back. (In an odd way, I'll know that I survived cancer when I die from something else.)

And what if I were living with metastatic cancer—that is, what if the cancer had spread to other parts of my body? Would I still be called a survivor? I'm not sure, but I wouldn't want anyone to think that I had lost or was losing. I would want people to think that I was living with cancer to the best of my ability.

Even the treatment for cancer is saddled with awkward language. Most people have heard chemotherapy referred to as poison. Chemotherapy is medicine. Any medicine—even aspirin—can be poisonous if taken incorrectly. Why should chemotherapy be singled out for its potential dangers and not for its potential benefits?

Casual conversations about cancer also cause people to speak in seemingly bizarre code. I often hear people refer to cancer as the Big C. Why don't we call diabetes the Big D or eczema the Big E?

Although cancer still makes us tongue-tied, we've made real progress in that we're trying to talk about it.

Fifty years ago, people often died of cancer without ever being told the diagnosis. (Of course, most people dying of cancer knew they were dying of cancer, whether they were told or not.) And today, more and more people are living—in every sense of the word—after a cancer diagnosis.

But we still have a ways to go in being comfortable with the language of cancer.

I'll be happy to discuss my cancer with you. Just don't ask about my battle. Ask about me.

The Look People Give You

A woman recently diagnosed with cancer who was aware of my newspaper column called me to say, "I wish you would tell people not to give me that look."

"What look?" I asked.

"The pity puss." (At first I thought she said "platypus," which I faintly recalled as being a weird-looking animal, and I wondered why on earth people were making platypus faces at her.)

Noting my momentary confusion, she continued, "Pity puss. Once I got diagnosed with cancer, people started looking at me as though I was a completely different person."

I knew the look she was referring to. When I was going through cancer treatment, people would look at me with solemn expressions and tilted heads as if they were looking deep into my soul. That look was always unsettling, especially when I was trying to eat lunch.

I asked other people with cancer if they've seen that look.

One woman told me that she knows the look, but it doesn't bother her because she knows it's coming from a place of caring. "Of course we have a list of things we want people to say or do, but cancer is emotionally loaded and scary. The solemn faces, teary eyeballs, and spiels about being brave aren't perfect gestures, but they show concern."

Another told me that she also knows the look, but what bothers her even more is the non-look. "Some people who used to make eye contact with me when saying 'good morning' now avert their eyes and hurry away fearing that a conversation might take place."

Once you've had cancer, you don't give "that look" when meeting someone else with cancer. One nurse told me, "It's like you guys with cancer have your own secret society." She's right. That's why spending time with others with cancer can be relaxing—because cancer isn't an elephant in the room. If people want to talk about cancer, fine. If people don't want to talk about cancer, that's fine too.

As I write this chapter, I'm afraid that I am making you so paranoid of making the wrong face or saying the wrong thing that your head might explode when encountering someone with cancer. Don't worry. What's in your heart is far more important than what you say or the expression on your face.

The most important lesson is to remember that your friend who now has cancer is the same person she was before she had cancer. If she liked hugs before, she'll like them now. If she was a private person before, she'll be a private person now.

If you're not sure what to say when you first talk with her after she's been diagnosed, try, "I'm so sorry."

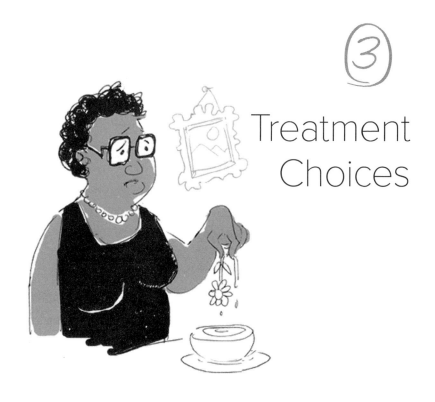

3
Treatment Choices

Alternative Cancer Therapies

People often fall into two camps regarding the usefulness of alternative cancer therapies. Some people are exuberant in their support of these therapies: "This dandelion soup is going to cure my cancer!" Others are completely dismissive. As is usually the case, a balanced perspective is more sensible than either extreme.

Alternative therapies include acupuncture, diet, exercise, massage, yoga, stress management, spiritual pursuits, aromatherapy, herbology, and many others. Sometimes they're referred to as complementary or integrative therapies.

The potential benefits and risks of any type of treatment—conventional or alternative—are especially significant with cancer because the stakes are so high. The choices a person makes can literally mean life or death.

Here's my take on the topic:

When people are diagnosed with cancer, they often feel a loss of control. Nearly anything you can do to regain some sense of control is understandable. Pursuing alternative treatment is an active process, and I think that's healthy.

Going through cancer is easier if one is part of a supportive community. I often see such communities emerge naturally from yoga classes, prayer circles, and exercise programs.

Don't force alternative modalities on others. The goal is to increase the patient's sense of control, not diminish it.

It's odd that some people think of good nutrition and exercise as alternative approaches to cancer care. They shouldn't be. Eating a well-balanced diet with less meat and more plant-based food is good for nearly everyone. And there's compelling evidence that exercise reduces the likelihood of recurrence for some cancers.

Some alternative approaches (e.g., massage) make a person feel better. As someone who's been through cancer treatment, I can say that anything that makes you feel better is a good thing.

Our organs and diseases don't exist in isolation. Maybe yoga won't directly affect your cancer, but it may affect your emotional well-being, which, in turn, can affect your cardiovascular system.

Don't begin radical lifestyle changes when beginning cancer treatment. There will be times when you'll need to sit on the couch and eat ice cream. That's OK. You need that rest and those calories.

Tell your doctors about your alternative approaches, even something that seems as benign as taking vitamins. This is especially true during chemotherapy. Antioxidants are usually good for people because they help keep cells alive, but chemotherapy is trying to kill cancer cells. The antioxidants can prevent the chemo from working. Other vitamins can affect how the body heals from surgery.

In sum, when thinking about alternative cancer modalities, the most important question isn't "Will this treatment cure my cancer?" Rather, the question to ask is, "Will this treatment contribute to my health and well-being?"

Alternative Practitioners

I recently asked a group of individuals with cancer about their experiences with alternative modalities and what advice they would have for alternative practitioners just beginning their careers. (It's interesting to note that nearly everyone in this group had pursued one or more such therapies.)

Many of their suggestions dealt with the need for nurturing and the creation of a healing space. Conventional cancer care focuses nearly exclusively on treatment. Healing is a different and largely unaddressed dimension that people yearn for.

Their favorite alternative practitioners were those who are comfortable with the language of Western medicine as well as their own areas of expertise. Many people diagnosed with cancer know a great deal about their disease and quickly assess if their practitioners are knowledgeable. In particular, most patients want to know how alternative therapies and mainstream treatment can work together.

Patients also appreciate when their practitioners—both conventional and alternative—are respectful of other approaches. They don't like their physicians to be dismissive of alternative modalities, nor do they like their alternative practitioners to be dismissive of Western medicine.

It's particularly important for patients and alternative practitioners to have a mutual understanding of what the alternative modalities are intended to achieve. What are the expectations and the boundaries of the practitioner's involvement?

The primary advice for alternative practitioners is the same advice I give to Western practitioners: Cancer patients are people. When you know them as individuals, you provide better care.

And cancer makes people especially vulnerable. They're scared when first diagnosed and then surprised to realize that their most basic questions often don't have clear answers. In my work at the Cancer Resource Center, I've learned that we often don't know the cause of a person's cancer or what the outcome will be if treatment is initiated.

As a result, cancer patients tend to develop relationships of trust with their care providers—both conventional and complementary. It is a shared journey and the best practitioners help light the path.

Clinical Trials

People diagnosed with cancer often wonder if they should participate in a clinical trial.

When someone asks for my opinion, I begin by saying that clinical trials are essential for the advancement of medicine. For example, one clinical trial found that women with early-stage breast cancer did just as well after a lumpectomy (followed by radiation) as did women who had a mastectomy. This finding greatly reduced the number of mastectomies that were being performed in this country and elsewhere.

That said, a clinical trial may or may not make the most sense for a specific individual. It's helpful to have a general understanding of the different types of clinical trials. A Phase 1 trial is a very small study to find out if a new treatment is safe. They aren't testing the effectiveness of the treatment against a particular disease, just its safety in humans. A Phase 2 trial is slightly larger and is used to determine if the new treatment seems to be effective in treating the disease under investigation.

If the Phase 2 trial is successful, a Phase 3 trial may be undertaken to determine how the new treatment compares to existing treatments. Is the treatment better, worse, or the same? These trials are much larger than Phase 1 or 2 trials, and patients are often recruited at multiple locations, including community hospitals. (Phase 1 and 2 trials usually take place only in major research institutions). The results of Phase 3 trials often change the standard of care.

Thus, clinical trials are good and are to be encouraged. Participating in a trial can also connect patients with professionals who are experts in their particular type of cancer.

But it is important to remember that the "new" treatment does not always prove to be better than the standard treatment. My advice for people considering a clinical trial is to talk with their oncologists as to which trials are available and the potential pros and cons of participating.

Here are some key points to consider:

* How effective is the standard treatment likely to be in your situation? In some cases, the standard treatment is highly effective and easily tolerated. In other cases, the standard treatment doesn't offer much hope. Knowing this information helps guide your decision-making.

* Is it a Phase 1, Phase 2, or Phase 3 trial? Phase 1 trials are riskier than Phase 2 trials, which are riskier than Phase 3 trials, but taking risks sometimes makes sense.

* If considering a trial, I'd ask the physician to compare the experimental treatment with the standard treatment. What are the potential benefits and what are the potential harms for each? Making this head-to-head comparison provides useful context.

* How convenient will it be for you to participate in the trial? While some trials are available locally, others require regular trips out of town. Some allow you to have blood tests and imaging (e.g., CT scans) performed locally. Others require that all tests be performed in the research hospital. Find out what's required by the trial that you're considering.

In sum, clinical trials are important, necessary, and worthwhile. Participating in a trial is altruistic because others with your disease will benefit. The benefit to you as an individual, however, depends on your specific situation. It's a good conversation to have with your oncologist.

Watching and Waiting

Most cancer diagnoses lead to treatment within a few weeks. For some cancers, however, the recommended course of action is to not treat the cancer unless it becomes worse.

Many of us have heard of "watching and waiting" being recommended for some men with prostate cancer, but it also happens with other cancers, including some forms of leukemia and lymphoma.

Danby, New York, resident Ben Hogben has a rare type of cancer known as hairy cell leukemia. Many people with this condition don't require treatment when first diagnosed, and some never require treatment. It's a matter of regular physical exams and closely monitoring lab results. Treatment is required only if blood counts fall below a certain level.

Most of us are conditioned to think that cancer needs to be attacked as aggressively and quickly as possible. Our whole vocabulary of cancer treatment is built on this approach—fighting cancer, battling cancer, defeating cancer. But, for Ben, the best treatment is no treatment—at least for now.

Can you imagine being told that you have cancer and that the recommended path is to keep a close eye on it? That has to be unsettling.

Ben's situation isn't unique, and it's made me realize that people with cancer who don't require immediate treatment can too easily fall between the cracks.

Those who are diagnosed with cancer and then go through

cancer treatment together very often form a tight bond. It's like the new freshman class entering college.

Those who get diagnosed with cancer but don't require treatment are mostly left to themselves to make sense of their uncertain status. It's like being wait-listed for college. They're in limbo and they're rarely connected with support programs. That's not a comfortable position for anyone.

Ben realizes that he has a cancer that generally isn't curable, but he notes that it is a *chronic* condition, not a *terminal* condition. He'll likely live several more decades.

He remembers being puzzled when his oncologist told him that he had the "good" leukemia. "What can be good about leukemia?" Ben thought to himself.

But he is doing well and is healthier than before through exercise and watching his diet. Sometimes knowing what we can't control makes us more aware of what we can control.

Too Little and Too Much Cancer Treatment

Although I firmly believe that everyone should be in control of their own treatment decisions, I have observed that some people seem to seek too little treatment when they are first diagnosed and other people seek too much treatment at the end of their lives.

Some people prefer to go the alternative route when they are first diagnosed. I'm a fan of many alternative treatments such as acupuncture, nutrition-based therapies, massage therapy, and other modalities. These treatments can complement conventional treatments and contribute to a person's well-being, but I worry when people say, "I'll try the alternative treatment first. If it doesn't work, I'll seek conventional treatment."

This is a concern because the best chance to cure many cancers is when they are first diagnosed. Delaying conventional treatment might lessen its potential effectiveness.

As I mentioned in the "Watching and Waiting" section just above, a decision might be made to not have *any* treatment when diagnosed with cancer. Perhaps the benefits of treatment are outweighed by the risks of treatment, or perhaps the patient just wants to take his or her chances with whatever may come. Not seeking treatment can be a reasonable approach.

I also hear people say, "Well, I'll have surgery, but I won't do chemotherapy or radiation because I'm philosophically opposed to them."

It's important to keep an open mind and not box yourself into a corner based on philosophy or generic understandings. Talk openly and honestly with your doctor about the potential benefits and potential harms of all of your treatment options so that you can make as informed a decision as possible.

While I see people sometimes *under*treat cancer when first diagnosed, I often see people *over*treat cancer toward the end of life. Once cancer has metastasized (spread to other parts of the body), cure becomes unlikely, but that doesn't necessarily mean it can't be treated. Treatment is designed to control the cancer and prevent it from getting worse. Each treatment that's tried eventually becomes ineffective because the cancer mutates or changes. When that happens, a new treatment is attempted.

Sometimes people think they have to keep treating their cancer—*fighting* their cancer—until the very end. They don't. Living a little longer when you feel miserable isn't a good trade-off in my mind.

You can ask your doctor how long a proposed new treatment will extend your life and what the side effects might be. The doctor can't answer with 100 percent certainty but should be able to provide some general guidelines as to what you can expect.

Decisions regarding cancer treatment are often difficult. In spite of what I've written in this chapter, these decisions aren't necessarily rational. Your life is more complicated than I or anyone else can imagine. Whatever you decide, know that you have the right to make those decisions and that those involved in your care will respect them. Further, know that you have the right to change your mind at any time. You are the one in control.

How Old Is Too Old to Treat Cancer?

The older you are, the more likely it is that you'll be diagnosed with cancer. The average age at diagnosis is now 67, and it's increasingly common for people in their late 80s and even older to consider cancer treatment.

Is this a good thing?

I think it's great when an 85-year-old says, "I want to aggressively treat my cancer. Give me chemo, give me whatever."

But I cringe when the relatives of an 85-year-old say, "We want to aggressively treat our father's cancer. Give him chemo, give him whatever."

The distinction, of course, is in who's making the request.

Treatment decisions are based on the likely benefits (e.g., extending one's life) and the likely costs (e.g., unpleasant side effects) of that treatment. Neither is known with certainty because there is so much individual variation, but doctors can provide some general guidance. They might say, "This treatment is relatively easy to tolerate and may extend your life for a few months, but no one knows for sure."

It's then up to the patient to decide if the treatment is worth pursuing. I'm very wary if I sense the family is more interested in aggressive treatment than is the patient. This is sometimes communicated quite subtly, "Oh Dad. I don't know if Mom can manage without you."

I also think some people pursue aggressive treatment because they "don't want to disappoint their doctors." Please don't worry about disappointing your doctors. They almost always have one more drug to try, and they're trained to keep trying.

I said I love it when an 85-year-old wants to aggressively treat his cancer. I also love it when an 85-year-old says, "I've had a good life and now I want to focus on the quality of my remaining life. Don't give me drugs to extend my life if those drugs will make me feel worse."

There may be less aggressive treatment options worth considering. In the United States, we tend to assume that the most aggressive treatment is always the "best" treatment. This isn't always the case, especially when factoring in quality of life. Perhaps there's another chemotherapy protocol that's easier to tolerate and still beneficial.

And be cautious if deciding on no additional treatment. Sometimes people say, "No more treatment," when they mean to say, "No more *life-extending* treatment." Radiation therapy is often given to reduce pain. Even some surgical procedures and chemotherapy treatments are designed not to extend life, but to provide comfort. Keep these options open.

Physicians and family members should also realize that age is not a good predictor of what others might decide. A few decades ago, some doctors automatically performed mastectomies on older patients with breast cancer (rather than consider less extensive surgery) because they assumed that older women wouldn't mind losing a breast. A word of advice I freely share with you: Never, ever make assumptions about anyone else's body parts.

Why Aren't They Doing More?

At the cancer resource center where I work, I sometimes get asked various versions of this question: "My father has advanced cancer, but they don't seem to be treating him very aggressively. Why aren't they doing surgery to remove the metastases in his lungs and liver?"

This is always a difficult question because the news is sometimes hard to absorb. When cancer metastasizes, or spreads, from its original location, the focus generally shifts from *curing* the cancer to *controlling* the cancer.

There are some exceptions. Relatively advanced testicular cancer is sometimes cured by aggressive chemotherapy and surgery. In other cancers, a few small metastatic tumors may be removed by surgery or radiation in the hopes of a cure.

In general, though, once the cancer spreads elsewhere in the body, surgery is not a viable option. Even if the surgeons remove all visible tumors, microscopic cancer cells have taken root in other organs. The analogy of trying to close the barn door after the horses have escaped is unfortunately apt.

The primary treatment for metastatic cancer is chemotherapy because chemo affects cells throughout the body. Many people respond well and their tumors shrink or stabilize. Stopping the progression of the disease is often the goal of chemotherapy for metastatic cancer.

Treatment for metastatic disease generally goes on for as long as the benefits of the treatment (extending one's life and/or reducing symptoms) outweigh the harm caused by the treatment (generally, the side effects of chemotherapy).

I facilitate a support group for people with advanced cancers. Many have been living with metastatic cancer for several years with a relatively good quality of life, often by receiving chemotherapy on an ongoing basis.

When someone asks me why the doctors aren't doing more to aggressively treating their father's cancer, I gently ask them what their father wants. I routinely find that patients come to peace with having a life-limiting illness before their loved ones do.

Remember, the most aggressive cancer treatment is not always the best cancer treatment. The person with cancer ultimately decides how much treatment is enough. The most fortunate patients make these decisions with the understanding and support of their loved ones. It's ok to ask those difficult questions. And it's ok to say, "Dad, I'm here for you if you want to continue treatment, and I'm here for you if you want to stop treatment. Just know that I'm here for you."

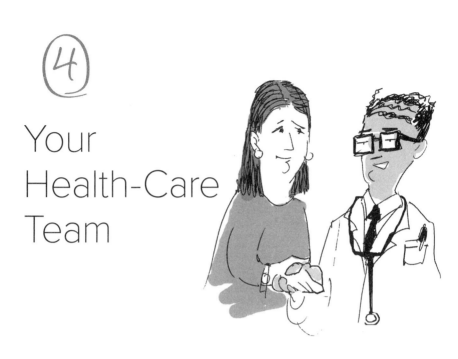

4

Your Health-Care Team

Communicating with Your Doctor

I'm always struck that some people diagnosed with cancer want to know absolutely everything about their disease while others just want to be told when to show up for treatment. Some people complain that their doctors give them too much information while others complain that their doctors give them too little.

Every doctor I've known will truthfully answer whatever questions are asked. The more difficult issue for doctors is what information to offer in the absence of questions. This is especially relevant when you are first diagnosed. Many people experience a brain freeze when they hear the words, "You have cancer," and are unable to ask any questions at all.

The basic information—diagnosis and suggested treatment—has to be shared, of course. But there's SO much information that could be discussed related to a cancer diagnosis. For example, should patients be told the survival statistics for their type of cancer?

Some patients diagnosed with a serious cancer want to know their chances of survival because it helps them plan their lives. Others don't want to know because they want only positive thinking around them. There's no right or wrong in this. What is important is for the doctor and patient to have a shared understanding of what works best for the patient.

Some doctors, of course, are better at sensing the patient's wishes than others. I encourage patients to tell their doctors how much or how little they want to know.

Another important time for clear communication is when a patient has metastatic or advanced cancer. Many of these patients can live for years with a good quality of life by receiving chemotherapy on an ongoing basis. There will come a time, though, when cancer cells mutate and become resistant to the current treatment and another treatment has to be initiated. When there are no more treatments to offer, the focus turns to comfort care, often through hospice.

Some people want to try every treatment option in order to extend their lives as long as possible. Others would rather focus on quality of life and not go through another round of chemotherapy. Again, what's important is for the patient to control these decisions.

Ending active treatment is a very personal decision and depends on the patient's condition and the treatment options. But I encourage patients to share their general mindset with their oncologist.

It's OK to say, "If I only have a few months to live, I'd rather spend those months in hospice." By saying that you're comfortable with hospice, it may allow the doctor to introduce hospice as a reasonable option earlier than he or she would have otherwise.

It's also OK to say, "My daughter is getting married next summer and I want to do everything possible to be at that wedding."

Like so much in life, the more that we share our wishes, the more likely it is that we'll get what we truly want.

Doctor–Patient Interactions

I spend much of my time helping seriously ill patients navigate the health-care system. As a result, I am constantly talking with patients about their interactions with doctors and other health professionals.

Although each encounter is unique, I am increasingly aware of some universal truths that contribute to good doctor–patient encounters. Not surprisingly, good encounters require a shared spirit of respect and communication.

I've found most providers to be committed to patient care and quality service. But all of us can benefit from gentle reminders from time to time.

Suggestions for doctors and other health professionals:

* Introduce yourself to new patients. This should be obvious, but it doesn't always happen.

* Listen for a while without interrupting. Get the big picture before filling in the details.

* Be kind.

* Remind yourself that patients newly diagnosed with a serious illness are scared. If you deal with sick people every day, it becomes routine. It's not routine for the new patient.

* Make a special effort to establish communication and a sense of partnership during the initial visit. Subsequent visits will benefit.

* Respect that patients may have beliefs—about health care, about life priorities, about whatever—that differ from your own.

* Recognize that medical care is costly for most people, even those with good insurance.

* Make good communication between patients and the entire office staff an ongoing priority. Few offices do this really well and every office could do it better.

Suggestions for patients:

* Recognize that you are not your doctor's only patient.

* Respect your doctor's time. If you have multiple questions, ask the most important questions first.

* Don't think of your doctor as the enemy. If you don't like your doctor, get a new one. Everyone will be happier.

* Be honest and open about your medical history and your present concerns. Don't make your doctor guess.

* Recognize that good health is largely your responsibility. Eat sensibly. Exercise. Don't smoke.

* Be reasonable. And be polite.

✳ Recognize that medicine is not a perfect science. A bad outcome does not mean bad care.

Good health care is a partnership. It's all about communication and respect. And it flows in both directions.

Chemo Nurses and Radiation Therapists

Chemotherapy nurses and radiation therapists provide much of the hands-on care to cancer patients. As a result, these professionals have a profound impact on the quality of care—and the quality of caring—that patients receive.

I attend a weekly breakfast club for guys who have had cancer. Last week, I asked them to describe the qualities in a chemo nurse or radiation therapist that made their weeks of treatment easier.

Most everyone said, in one way or another, "They saw me as a person, not just as a patient."

One man continued, "They took the time to get to know me as an individual. I could tell that I wasn't just a body part or type of cancer that needed attention. That made a huge difference to me."

When a person is first diagnosed with cancer, there's often a sense that life is out of control. The best nurses and therapists provide a sense of quiet calm and say, in words and action, "We'll get you through this." Patients begin to relax.

Sometimes it is a matter of recognizing and acknowledging the patient's anxiety. New cancer patients feel especially raw and vulnerable. The best caregivers put patients at ease by witnessing that fear and not dismissing it.

Some professionals seem to have an almost telepathic sense when things aren't right. They pick up subtle cues from the patient's body language and facial expressions and then gently probe for more information.

The potential side effects of cancer treatment are overwhelming. Good nurses and therapists clearly explain what's to be expected, what's unusual, and when to call for help. That sounds simple, but it isn't because every patient is so different. Discussions need to be tailored to the patient's level of understanding and style of learning. And family members need to be involved as well.

Warmth of spirit and good humor are also essential for providing cancer care. No one wants a crabby nurse or therapist. I'm constantly amazed at how much humor is present in oncology. I think people relish laughter when sadness is never far away.

At the end of treatment, patients invariably say, "I'm going to miss those guys." While providing complex treatment, the nurses and therapists provided security, comfort, and kindness. And they became friends.

The Art and Science of Oncology

I suspect most people—and many health professionals—think of treating cancer patients as being especially challenging. Some of those challenges are fairly obvious—people with cancer are often very sick, death sometimes looms as a possible outcome, and everyone in the waiting room is scared.

Other challenges are less obvious. A cancer diagnosis affects the entire family. Family members have questions and opinions, and family dynamics (both good and bad) are amplified. It's not unusual for the patient to be the calmest person in the room.

Treating cancer patients requires what I think of as compartmentalization. The professional has to be completely present with each patient and not be thinking about the previous patient or the next one. This is a skill that doesn't come naturally to most of us. This is especially difficult in oncology because some patients are doing great, some are dying, and others are living in a world of uncertainty. The gamut of human emotions can be witnessed in a single morning.

Another challenge is responding to questions that don't have definitive answers. Patients often want to know what the future holds for them. Statistics can provide general guides, but no one knows for sure how an individual will respond to a particular treatment or if their cancer will return. By its very nature, cancer is unpredictable.

Science is the starting point of cancer care, but there is an art to applying that science to each patient. This art is based on clinical experience, judgment, and intuition. Patients don't always fit into neat little boxes with obvious choices for the best treatment.

The importance of communication can't be overstated. Patients need to understand their treatment options and the probable benefits and risks of pursuing those options. Try explaining anything to people of differing ages, education levels, and cultural values. Then try it when those people are scared and part of what needs to be explained is uncertain. It isn't easy.

I want to make special mention of chemotherapy nurses and radiation therapists who work with cancer patients. In addition to providing care, they often become the grounding force that keeps the patient together during these difficult months. Something as simple as a calming hand on the shoulder can make a remarkable difference. Sometimes the patient uses the nurses and therapists as relief valves—patients can say things that they can't say to their family members. In some ways, the therapy room is a safe place because the word "cancer" doesn't make anyone flinch.

There are inevitable times of sadness when working with cancer patients. People die, sometimes unexpectedly. And there are also times of happiness when people do well and return to their lives, cured of what was once an incurable disease.

What I've come to realize is that there is always something that can be done to help a person with cancer. Even if the disease can't be cured, a patient's quality of life can be affected in a positive manner. It's not a profession for everyone. But I'm happy that so many good people have chosen it.

5

Caring for Yourself During Treatment

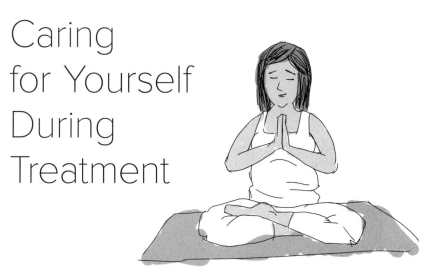

Keeping Yourself in Balance

Yesterday afternoon, a woman about to begin chemotherapy came into my office and asked, "What advice do you have to help me get through my treatment?" I've been asked this question in various forms hundreds of times. I now realize that the answer boils down to this: "Keep things in balance."

It's all about being reasonable. I hesitate to make reference to "common sense," because common sense is gained through experience and cancer is new to everyone the first time through.

Here are some examples:

Activity level

I've known some patients to remain flat on their backs throughout months of chemotherapy while others push themselves to compete in athletic events the day after treatment. In general, moderate activity is good and either extreme is counterproductive. Too little activity makes fatigue worse, and too much activity drains energy when it's needed for healing. Walking is often more beneficial than either sitting or running.

Information-seeking

Some people want to know everything about their cancer and its treatment, while others want to know as little as possible. Information is almost always helpful, especially when it helps people understand what to expect. For example, you don't want to be surprised when your hair falls out. But too much information can be as harmful as too little information. I've seen people become paralyzed from studying long lists of potential side effects or from getting fifth and sixth medical opinions.

Calling the doctor

Cancer treatment invariably causes side effects. Some side effects are serious and others are more of a nuisance. At one extreme are patients who call the doctor's office ten times a day. At the other extreme are people who never call, even if experiencing fever, pain, or other serious problems. Nurses are great at explaining which side effects are routine and expected, and which ones require attention that day. Take their instructions to heart.

Cancer 24/7

Some patients focus on their cancer 24 hours a day. It's all they talk and think about. Other patients never discuss their cancer and essentially deny that they have it, even in the midst of treatment. One can acknowledge cancer and deal with it, but also take a break from it from time to time. Go out to a movie or dinner and talk about anything but cancer for a few hours.

Sense of control

Cancer is unpredictable and we often lose our sense of control. During treatment, patients are reassured that problems will be addressed if and when they occur. That seems reactive rather than proactive and it makes people uneasy. Sometimes, though, patients (and their families) just need to, well, chill. But it's a mistake to become overly passive and not control what can be controlled. Most patients can control how they spend their time and how they take care of themselves. One man put it like this, "I'm letting my doctors work on the cancer. I'm working on making my body healthier."

Every situation and every person is different, so there are no hard and fast rules for all of this. But I think the concepts of balance and moderation during cancer treatment are useful. When people are at one extreme or the other, they tend to experience more problems and more stress. Cancer is never easy, but keeping yourself in balance will make it more manageable.

Cancer-Related Anxiety

The days following a cancer diagnosis are almost always filled with anxiety. (I have, however, talked with a few people who were relieved when they were diagnosed. They instinctively knew that they had cancer, and getting the diagnosis brought them peace of mind and allowed them to move forward.)

But most people who are newly diagnosed wake up with worried thoughts about cancer and go to sleep with worried thoughts about cancer. And quite a few toss and turn more than they actually sleep. Managing this anxiety is important because anxiety causes people to make poor treatment decisions.

Sometimes the anxiety causes individuals to be overly aggressive in their treatment. Some people request the most extensive treatment possible even though more modest treatment (or no treatment) may be just as effective. Undergoing the most aggressive treatment may be appropriate and entirely reasonable, but anxiety shouldn't be the deciding factor.

Anxiety causes other people to become paralyzed. They don't make treatment decisions on a timely basis because they think about every "what if" possibility. What if the radiation therapy causes some other form of cancer 20 years from now? What if a new and better treatment is just around the corner?

Treatment decisions are difficult for nearly everyone because there is always some degree of uncertainty. There are no guarantees.

A critical factor is the relationship between you and your doctor. If you trust your doctor, you'll be less anxious. If you don't trust your doctor, get a new one.

Besides having trust in your physicians, what can you do to reduce anxiety?

* When people are wrestling with treatment decisions, I encourage them to write down a list of reasons to do a particular treatment and a list of the reasons not to do

that treatment. People who are overly anxious tend to ask the same questions over and over again. If they prepare a list of pros and cons and then refer to that list, they're less likely to spin around in a thousand directions.

* Physical exercise helps clear one's thinking. Activities such as yoga often bring a sense of centering, stillness, and clarity. And there are programs such as Mindfulness-Based Stress Reduction that specifically help people recognize and cope with the stress that often accompanies serious illness.

* Getting a good night's sleep is underappreciated. If you are not sleeping well because of anxiety, you're probably not making thoughtful decisions. Sleeping pills and anti-anxiety medication are sometimes helpful and appropriate in dealing with the stress of a new cancer diagnosis. Talk with your physician about what makes sense for you.

Experiencing anxiety when diagnosed with cancer is normal. But managing that anxiety is essential for making clear-headed decisions.

Cancer and Depression

Many people who have cancer go through a period of depression. It can happen during treatment or many months or even years later. What especially concerns me is that many cancer patients who are depressed never report their depression to their doctors.

There are many phrases that people use to describe depression: a lack of energy, not enjoying what one used to enjoy, not wanting to get out of bed.

The obvious reason for treating depression is that most people benefit from it. They feel better with medication and/or talk therapy. It improves their quality of life, not to mention the quality of the lives of those around them.

A less obvious reason, but one that is critically important for those with cancer, is that people who are depressed tend to be poor decision-makers. Sometimes they make decisions they wouldn't have made had they been more clear-headed. Other times, they can't seem to decide anything and find themselves spinning in circles.

Everyone with cancer has decisions to make. Should the cancer be treated? Which kind of treatment makes the most sense? Where should they go for treatment? Making these decisions when depressed is difficult.

When patients tell me that they're depressed, I always ask if they've told this to their physician. Quite often, the answer is no. They may feel that depression is "normal" given a cancer diagnosis. Or they feel that they can tough it out. Some say that they don't want to take any more pills.

I respond by saying that depression after a cancer diagnosis is common, but that doesn't make it normal. At the very least, they should discuss their emotional well-being with their oncologist or primary-care physician. Many people need treatment for only a few months in order to adjust to the changes that accompany a serious illness. Not treating the depression may also be a reasonable approach for some people, but this decision should be made in consultation with your physician.

Depression is also closely associated with anxiety, which independently affects people's ability to make clear and thoughtful decisions. Treating depression often helps the anxiety and vice-versa.

Getting emotional help following a cancer diagnosis is not a sign of weakness but of strength. Cancer often causes people to feel like their lives are out of control. Seeking treatment for depression and anxiety is an important first step in regaining that control.

More than Tired

When people think about the side effects of cancer treatment, they usually think about hair loss (which is common with some types of chemotherapy) and nausea (which is not nearly as common as it used to be). In my mind, though, fatigue is the side effect of cancer treatment that's both most universal and least appreciated.

Fatigue is different from simply being tired. People often describe it as a complete loss of energy. I hear the phrases "dead tired" or "bone tired" all of the time. Washing the dishes can seem like climbing Mount Everest. And people often wake up in the morning feeling just as depleted. Fatigue is more than a nuisance—it can completely disrupt one's life.

Some causes of cancer-related fatigue are organic and respond well to treatment. Anemia, for example, is sometimes caused by chemotherapy. If people don't have enough red blood cells, they won't feel very peppy. Anemia can be treated.

Sometimes fatigue is caused by simply not eating enough. Treatment (and cancer itself) can affect a person's appetite or ability to swallow. Nutritionists can help identify foods and supplements that are both palatable and provide enough calories. Medication can be used to stimulate a person's appetite if it continues to be a problem.

Sleep is often disrupted during cancer treatment. A person's life rhythms get out of whack—they go to bed at odd hours, nap during the day, and worry at regular intervals. The medications themselves can affect sleep cycles. A good night's sleep restores both a person's body and emotions. If sleep is a problem, talk with your doctor about medication and/or other solutions.

Depression is common for many people with cancer and depression can independently affect sleep, appetite, and energy. Many cancer patients have found that treatment for depression addresses their fatigue as well.

For many, the cause of fatigue is the lack of activity. It's easy to become out of shape after months of surgery, chemo, and radiation. It's a vicious cycle in that fatigue can cause one to stay on the couch, which, in turn, causes more fatigue. Gentle exercise, such as walking, is almost always helpful.

Even when the fatigue can't be "fixed," it can be managed. One nurse tells her patients that it's like beginning each day with $100 in their energy bank. Once it's gone for the day, it's gone, so they need to prioritize their activities. At the top of the list are things that have to get done as well as those things that provide the greatest pleasure. Other activities can wait or friends can be called in to help with the dishes or shop for groceries. Friends who want to help are often delighted to have concrete tasks assigned.

Cancer-related fatigue is just beginning to receive the attention it deserves. Just as pain assessment has become a standardized and regular component of medical care, fatigue assessment is entering the realm of routine cancer care. One survey of cancer patients found that most experienced fatigue, but few discussed it with their physicians. I hope this soon changes. Just like pain, fatigue can be overwhelming and debilitating. It can and should be addressed as a matter of course.

Chemobrain

Some people report memory loss, slower mental processing speed, and other cognitive changes after chemotherapy. Anyone who has been in a cancer support group has heard these symptoms described as chemobrain, but only recently have researchers and clinicians given it much attention. "Chemobrain" turns out to be a complicated issue because so many factors may be involved.

Nearly every cancer patient experiences fatigue and stress, and a significant number report some degree of depression, all of which can affect a person's memory and ability to think clearly. And cancer is most common in individuals over the age of 65, a time when cognitive changes might appear independently of cancer or its treatment. Measuring cognitive changes specifically caused by chemotherapy is difficult.

I had chemotherapy several years ago, and I experienced what I consider to be chemobrain. It didn't affect my day-to-day functioning, but it did seem to hamper my ability to kick my brain into its highest gear. For a college professor—which I was at the time—losing high gear can be a serious problem. Fortunately, the symptoms disappeared in a few months as they do for most people. In some cases, though, chemobrain seems to linger on for years.

So what does this all mean for someone just now diagnosed with cancer? Here's my take:

* Realize that most people undergoing chemotherapy do not experience cognitive problems. If your brain seems fuzzy when you're getting cancer treatment, report these symptoms to your doctor. Some problems can be corrected by changing medications or some other relatively easy fix.

* If you feel depressed, share that with your doctor. Depression is treatable.

* Exercise during treatment is often helpful. Aerobic activity can clear your mind and make you feel more alert.

In sum, there is a growing recognition that cognitive changes sometime occur as a result of cancer and its treatment, but we don't know exactly why it happens or who is at greatest risk. In general, these changes are transient and manageable, but we're just beginning to understand the scope of the problem and what to do about it.

The Uncertainty of Cancer

Before you get diagnosed with cancer, you assume that it will be an unpleasant experience, but one that is pretty straightforward.

One might think, "I have this type of cancer, so I will get that type of treatment." Like getting a hernia fixed, only more serious. But cancer is filled with uncertainty, and hardly anyone is prepared for it.

Patients often ask: Why did I get cancer? Will I be cured? Which side effects will I experience? Which treatment is best?

Oncologists often respond to these questions by saying, "I don't know." They aren't hiding anything—they really don't know. No one does.

Uncertainty can occur because there's so much variation in how individuals respond to treatment.

You can give two people the exact same chemotherapy drugs—one will sail through without any problems and the other will feel awful every single day.

One person will be cured by a particular treatment and another individual with the same diagnosis will have a recurrence within a few months.

Sometimes uncertainty exists because there's no data that specifically answers the question. For example, I'm a guy with breast cancer. There isn't much research on treating male breast cancer, so it's generally assumed that what works for postmenopausal women will work for me, too.

Entirely reasonable, but not altogether reassuring.

Even common cancers are fraught with uncertainty. Men with prostate cancer may be given the options of surgery, radiation, or watchful waiting. Sometimes the best option for a particular patient is clear. Other times, it's a complete toss-up.

Uncertainty continues after treatment is completed. The big question for most people is whether the cancer will return.

As someone who has had cancer, let me say that this uncertainty really sucks.

A change in perspective can be positive.

I was walking my dog on a cloudy Ithaca day when she came across a ray of sunlight hitting the sidewalk. She immediately sat down, closed her eyes, and relished the pure joy of sitting in the sun. That image of her living purely in the moment stays with me. And my cancer, as cancers go, was pretty good. That is, my risk of a recurrence is low, especially now that several years have passed. But I no longer feel invincible. Of course, you don't have to have cancer to face uncertainty. It's part of the human experience.

Several people have said to me, "Too bad you got cancer, but life is uncertain for everyone. I could be hit by a bus tomorrow." (I'm never sure how to respond to this comment. "God willing" seems a bit awkward.)

Cancer and uncertainty do go hand-in-hand. It's good in some ways and bad in others. Like many other realities, it just is and we go forward the best we can.

Uncertainty and Commitments

Being diagnosed with cancer changes one's sense of the future. You wonder if you'll die from cancer and, if so, when.

There's rarely a definite answer to these questions, so uncertainty becomes an unwanted companion. For the most part, this uncertainty is an abstraction floating around in the back of your head, but it becomes concrete at unexpected times.

For me, it became real when I thought about investing the money in my retirement account. Before cancer, I assumed that I would eventually enjoy many years of healthy retirement. After cancer, I wasn't so sure that I would even reach retirement age. Investing for the long-term suddenly seemed risky.

My cancer hasn't returned, and, although there's a slight risk of a recurrence, I'm again working on the assumption that I'll enjoy many years of retirement. But other people with cancer aren't so fortunate.

A woman in treatment asked me a blunt question: "How can I make commitments when I'm dealing with a crappy diagnosis?"

She went on, "It's hard for me to commit to doing something next week because I don't know how I'll feel. And bigger commitments—like starting a new relationship or a new job—seem impossible."

She was asking the question rhetorically, but I've been thinking about it ever since. I wish I had a simple answer.

I do know that living with uncertainty is easier if you're surrounded by people who understand and accept that uncertainty. They are there for you no matter what. It's so much more difficult without that support.

At a recent cancer support group, Rev. Tim Dean, Chaplain at Cayuga Medical Center, said that serious illness often makes us more authentic. Perhaps that's why making commitments is sometimes more difficult when cancer is present. The commitments need to be honest and authentic. There's not much pretense when you're bald from chemotherapy.

But perhaps that is some of the good that can emerge from the bad of cancer. When someone is with you through cancer, or even after cancer, they are with you all the way.

The Transitions of Cancer

My job is to listen to people affected by cancer and to help them however I can. With experience, I've come to understand that the periods of greatest stress and emotional turmoil are often predictable. When people come to my office, they're usually at one of four periods of transition.

The first transition is the short time between being diagnosed with cancer and beginning treatment. People have to wrap their heads around a potentially life-threatening illness, and they're typically overwhelmed with information and advice. They need to decide which treatment, if any, to pursue and are wondering if they should get a second or third opinion. Critical decisions have to be made when no one can say for sure which decision will turn out to be the "correct" one. High levels of stress during this phase are common.

The second transition is at the end of treatment. This seems counterintuitive, but most people are scared when they complete their last radiation therapy or chemo session. It's often described as leaving the safety of the cocoon. People miss seeing their health professionals on a regular basis, and they worry about the cancer returning. One's imagination goes into overdrive. A headache isn't just a headache, it's a brain tumor. And it takes more time than expected to bounce back and resume one's previous life.

The first two transitions are almost universal. The next two occur only if cancer returns.

The third transition is at the time of a recurrence. When cancer returns, the focus of treatment generally shifts from curing the cancer to controlling the cancer. That's a huge mental adjustment. As a friend recently said to me, "When I was first diagnosed with cancer, it was a bump in the road in my life. Now, I have advanced cancer and it IS the road in my life."

The fourth transition occurs when people with advanced cancer get worse. They have to decide if they want to keep trying new treatments with the hope of living longer, or if they'd rather stop active treatment and focus on comfort and quality of life through hospice.

Living with cancer is never a straight line, but these four periods of transition are the times of greatest anxiety and uncertainty. If people with cancer anticipate these periods, perhaps the transitions will be a little less difficult. And if their loved ones are aware of the transitions, perhaps they will know when to be most available, most attentive, and most supportive.

How You Feel and How You Look

Cancer is a weird disease because you can have it and not be sick. Or you can look pretty good when you *are* sick. This is confusing for our friends who are trying to say or do the right thing. It can be just as confusing for those of us with cancer.

When I was first diagnosed with breast cancer, I didn't feel sick at all. It was odd to plan surgery and chemotherapy when I felt in perfect health.

But when I was going through chemotherapy a few months later, I became irritated when people told me that I looked good. I didn't feel so good, and I wanted people to somehow recognize that. Of course, I didn't want people to tell me that I looked like crap, either.

So, what should friends and family say to be helpful? I've brought this up at support groups and there's never a consensus. Everyone seems to have a different opinion. In fact, most everyone seems to have more than one opinion, and those opinions aren't necessarily consistent or rational. How can friends know what to say if those of us with cancer don't know what we want to hear?

But then I heard a colleague, Kerry Quinn, gently ask a patient, "Do you feel as good as you look?"

I realized that this was a perfect question because it doesn't assume anything. It simply asks the patient if how they feel on the inside matches how they look on the outside.

When asked, patients usually pause and reflect. And then they begin to talk.

Cancer
As a Marathon

Chris LaVallee ran a 7-day, 155-mile race in the Australian wilderness to raise funds for the Cancer Resource Center of the Finger Lakes.

I heard him describe the race and his training and then answer questions from an audience of supporters. One asked, "How do you keep going mentally when your body is exhausted?"

As Chris began to answer, I realized that distance running is a perfect metaphor for cancer treatment.

Anyone who has had cancer can tell you that it's a marathon and not a sprint. At the starting line, everyone is pumped up because of the cheering crowd and the uncertainty of what lies ahead. The challenge is when the starting line is far behind and the finish line isn't yet in sight. Physical and mental fatigue can be overwhelming.

Distance runners expect this fatigue and train for it. Their coaches prepare them to "run through it."

People with cancer rarely have the opportunity to train before beginning treatment. And they're likely to be more concerned about losing their hair, throwing up, and dying than about fatigue.

But they're surprised to find that fatigue is often the most disruptive side effect of treatment. There's the physical fatigue that sometimes makes getting out of bed a challenge. And then there's the mental fatigue. If the first four cycles of chemotherapy knocked you on your butt, you know the fifth cycle won't be any easier.

Just as runners appreciate those who cheer them on far into the race, people with cancer especially appreciate their supporters who cheer them on far into treatment. There's always a crowd at the starting line and the finish line. We most remember the solitary cheerleader who gives us a lift when we most need it.

Many people with early cancer receive chemotherapy and/or radiation for a set period of time to reduce the risk of a recurrence. There's a clear finish line.

But people with more advanced cancers often receive chemotherapy on an ongoing basis to keep their cancers under control. This is like being a distance runner in a long race without a clear finish line. They just keep running. I really admire their, well, athleticism.

Let's all give a cheer to marathon runners like Chris. And let's cheer as well for our family members, friends, and neighbors as they face the challenges of cancer with strength and perseverance.

Cancer and Relationships

Single with Cancer

For a day or two following chemotherapy, most people camp out on the couch and do nothing more strenuous than watch TV or flip through magazines.

Loved ones bring glasses of water, cups of tea, and small snacks to lift the patient's spirits and provide nourishment.

If you're single, going through cancer treatment can be especially challenging. If you don't get off the couch to fetch your own water, you may go thirsty.

You also worry about who's going to drive you to doctor appointments, relay information to relatives and friends, do the grocery shopping, and walk the dog.

There are financial issues: If you can't work, you don't get paid. Even short-term absences from work can be difficult. Your income may go down just as your expenses go up. There's no cushion of a second income or a spouse's health insurance.

And who's going to be with you in those dark moments when everyone else goes home? It's scary when it's quiet and your mind inevitably wanders to those "what if" questions.

Perhaps you're in a new romantic relationship or simply looking forward to future relationships. Cancer tends to complicate all of this. Potential changes in body image, fertility, and even life expectancy can be difficult subjects to navigate.

But all is not gloom. People are remarkably resilient, and that is certainly true for most single people with cancer.

Some single people I know actually prefer going through cancer treatment alone. They like having the freedom to focus strictly on their own needs and "not putting on a happy face for others."

And, of course, not every marriage or partnership is a good one. Having an unsupportive partner during cancer treatment might well be worse than having no partner at all.

Although cancer can complicate new relationships, it can be a positive force as well. I've seen several relationships (both romantic and otherwise) take root during and after cancer treatment. When you have cancer, you tend to worry less about the small stuff and appreciate the good that's around you.

Often the good around you comes in the form of dear friends who step up and support you in your journey.

But when there's no one to help fetch that glass of water, you do it yourself. And you continue to move forward.

Postcancer Relationships

It can be a challenge to begin a new relationship after having had cancer. We usually think about this from the perspective of the person with cancer, but what about the other partner in a new relationship—the one without cancer?

One woman put it this way: "I feel like cancer is a member of his family. I want to understand and help, but he never wants to talk about it."

This reminds me of those old movies in which the newcomer to the household realizes there's a mysterious person living in the attic. This person is never mentioned even though his footsteps are heard from time to time. The newcomer is concerned and curious, but it's clear that questions aren't welcomed.

That's not a comfortable situation in the movies or in real life.

I encourage the partner with cancer to be as open as possible. Some people want to compartmentalize their cancer experience and not think about it again. That doesn't work well if there's a new partner. Like it or not, cancer is part of your life, so share it.

And I encourage the partner without cancer to ask questions. If your partner doesn't want to answer those questions just then, try to schedule a time to sit down and talk it through.

Talking about cancer is scary, but not talking about cancer is even scarier.

New relationships after cancer can be challenging even with good communication.

When a person goes through cancer with a partner, it's generally a shared experience. Together, they learn the language of cancer and mutually understand what's been done and what the future holds. If the relationship develops after the cancer diagnosis and treatment, the partner without cancer needs to catch up.

For some new couples, the cancer is mostly a distant memory that has little impact. Perhaps a scar and an annual checkup are the only reminders.

For other couples, cancer is a day-to-day presence. Some cancers require ongoing treatment. Even cancers that are presumably cured can have significant aftereffects: changes in body image, colostomies, sexual difficulties, infertility, fatigue. These are real challenges to a new relationship.

I love meeting couples who fall in love in spite of these challenges. If you can work together through cancer, you can work together through anything.

And having had cancer is not all bad. People who have been through serious illness don't take much for granted.

Life doesn't have to be perfect to be good.

When a Partner Is in Denial

I recently spoke with a woman who was stressed because her husband has cancer and he seemed to be in denial over the seriousness of his situation.

What was especially upsetting to her was that he didn't want to address any end-of-life issues like drafting a will.

I've been mulling this over ever since. What happens when a couple faces cancer and they aren't on the same page?

It's sometimes a matter of perspective. Is the glass half full or half empty? With a particular cancer, the chance of surviving might be 80 percent. On the other hand, the chance of dying is 20 percent. Different people focus on different numbers.

It can also be a function of timing. Absorbing a diagnosis of cancer doesn't happen overnight, and people have to do it at their own pace. Your partner won't necessarily process the news and accompanying emotions on your timetable.

And realize that denial might be a useful coping strategy in the short term. It's how your partner can get through the next few weeks without falling apart.

Here are a few recommendations:

* It is almost always helpful for a couple to attend medical appointments together so they can hear the same news at the same time. It's hard to be in synch emotionally if you aren't working from the same set of facts.

* Be patient with your partner. Listen without judgment.

* At the same time, recognize and address your own needs. Joining a support group can provide an emotional outlet and a chance to connect with others in similar situations.

* Too much about cancer is uncertain and uncontrollable, so control what you can control. Everyone should have a will and a health-care proxy. Take care of them so there are fewer things to worry about. If your spouse balks, say that it's important for your peace of mind and then take the initiative in making the arrangements.

Sometimes the person in denial is the individual with cancer. Just as often, it's the partner of the person with cancer who's the one in denial. Either way, the principles of being patient and supportive of your partner while addressing your own needs work equally well.

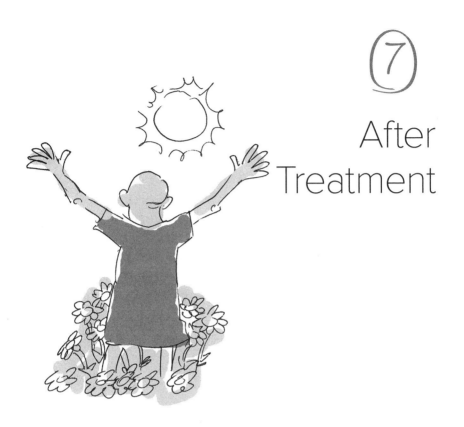

7

After Treatment

The Posttreatment Blahs

For many people, the months following cancer treatment are more difficult than the treatment itself.

During treatment, your "job" is to be in treatment. You're busy with appointments and you see the same doctors and nurses almost every week. At the same time, friends bring you meals, family members take on extra duties, and you're left to focus on getting better.

Then you have your last radiation therapy treatment or chemotherapy session. You get hugs and congratulatory handshakes. There's an expectation that everything in your life will suddenly revert back to normal.

Let me pop that bubble: Everything doesn't return to normal right away. You might even wonder, "Is my *new* normal the same as my *old* normal?" Your body is tired. Your brain is muddled. You're worried that the cancer will come back. And you miss the safe cocoon of your chemo nurses and radiation therapists.

What makes it especially hard is that the people around you sometimes expect you to bounce back almost immediately. While they were happy to help you during treatment, they now see you as recovered and expect you to carry your old load.

The posttreatment blahs are so common that I try to prepare people for them in advance. This is what I suggest:

* Expect a post-treatment slump. Rather than being a time of celebration, the last treatment is sometimes the beginning of a funk. If you expect that funk, it won't be so difficult.

* Realize that recovery is not a straight line. You'll feel better one day but worse the next. That's normal.

* Expect recovery to take several months. Some people say that the recovery phase takes as long as the treatment phase. It took me a full year following chemotherapy to really feel like myself again.

* Expect to be acutely aware of every ache and pain and immediately think the worst. Every headache is an ominous sign of a brain tumor instead of just a normal headache. Every cough is a lung metastasis instead of a normal

cold. These worries become even more pronounced before doctor visits and tests. You scan your body for the slightest indication of anything bad. Everyone goes through this.

* Realize that cancer will continue to be front and center in your life for several more months. It's what you think about in the morning, at night, and throughout the day. But this fades with time. The second year after treatment is much easier than the first year after treatment.

* Expect your family and friends to have less time to sit with you and listen to your concerns about living with cancer. They're eager to get back to normal as quickly as possible. There's a good chance that you still want to process what you've been through. Joining a support group or speaking with a therapist can be especially helpful during this transition phase.

Most of all, be patient with those around you and especially with yourself.

Don't Look Back

It is easy to second-guess yourself when you have cancer. It can take many forms:

* I wouldn't have cancer if I had taken better care of myself.

* I should have gone to the doctor sooner.

* I should have chosen Treatment B instead of Treatment A.

* I should have chosen "watchful waiting" instead of aggressive treatment.

Nearly everyone with cancer wonders if they would be better off had they made different decisions somewhere along the line.

Most of us would have led healthier lives had we known that cancer was looming in our futures. But there's no guarantee that it would have made any difference. Many cancers occur seemingly at random, even to those who have led the healthiest of lifestyles.

Treatment decisions have to be made based on the information that's available and your sense of what is best for you. That's the best that we can do.

If your treatment caused problems, you're likely to compare it to an idealized version of other treatment options, but those treatments may have caused similar or even worse problems for you.

Our knowledge is constantly evolving. When I had my mastectomy for breast cancer in 1996, I had an axillary node dissection in which several of the lymph nodes under my arm were removed. Had I been diagnosed a year later, I would have had a less invasive procedure known as a sentinel lymph node dissection in which fewer lymph nodes are removed. The treatment you received will always be replaced by better treatments.

We also evolve as individuals. The priorities we had ten years ago aren't necessarily the priorities we have today. Making a different decision today doesn't mean that a decision made in the past was incorrect.

It's also important to focus your energies on where they can make a difference. You may be able to reduce your risk of a cancer recurrence by what you do today and tomorrow. You can't change the past.

Everyone with cancer wonders "what if…?" from time to time, but don't ask yourself that question too often. We need to let go and move forward.

Cancer As a Chronic Disease

Until recently, people have undergone cancer treatment with the goal of ridding the body of cancer. Sometimes the treatment worked and the cancer went away, either temporarily (a remission) or permanently (a cure). If the treatment did not work, the cancer generally got worse and the person died. Success or failure.

Today, a new category of cancer care is emerging: the management of cancer as a chronic disease. Some cancers aren't curable, but they're controllable, with a good quality of life, for years or even decades.

Living with cancer as a chronic disease is made possible, in part, by the availability of new chemotherapy drugs. In the past, only one treatment may have been available for a particular type of cancer. If that stopped working (or never worked), there were no other tools to try. Today, when Treatment A stops working, the person might be switched to Treatment B, and later to Treatment C. (You might hear this referred to as first-line treatment, second-line treatment, and so forth.)

I regularly visit with people when they are at the hospital receiving chemotherapy. Most come for a period of three or four months, but a few come in for chemo week after week and month after month. You'd expect these "frequent fliers" to be really sick, but many look good and seem remarkably upbeat. I'm always reminded of the television show *Cheers*. I half expect Norm to walk in and plop himself into a chemo chair as nurses and other patients in the chemotherapy suite call out his name.

People are able to tolerate long-term chemo because many of the newest drugs have fewer side effects than traditional chemotherapy drugs, and the side effects from all types of chemo are now managed better than ever before. The awful nausea that accompanied chemotherapy a generation ago is now quite rare.

I also think that people in long-term treatment become quite adept at setting priorities and managing their time. There's a rhythm to chemotherapy, and people know when they'll feel good and when they won't. The good times are reserved for what's most important and/or what's most enjoyable.

People in treatment also relish simply feeling good. When you're healthy, you take feeling good for granted. When you're sick, feeling good is a gift like the first day of spring.

Thinking of cancer as a chronic disease is new and progress is incremental. Some cancers have effective second- and third-line treatments available while others don't. And all cancers have the ability to mutate and become resistant to every tool in the oncologist's toolbox. There is still plenty of uncertainty. But for many people with advanced cancers, a new era of treatment is emerging.

The absence of a cure is not the absence of hope.

Survivor's Guilt

People going through cancer treatment at the same time often form their own peer group. They see each other in chemo, in radiation, and in various support groups. The fortunate ones do well, but they often feel guilty when others in their cohort succumb to the disease.

Survivor's guilt is a well-known phenomenon, but it's usually thought of in the context of war, disasters, and other catastrophic events. Why does one person live when others perish?

With cancer, the emergence of survivor's guilt is a slower, more-subtle process. There's a gradual realization that many of the people who once gathered together for a support group are no longer living.

Sometimes the loss is expected. Some cancers clearly have poorer prognoses than others. But sometimes it seems completely arbitrary, especially when a person's "cancer buddies" are those with the same cancer.

I'm not a fan of using military metaphors when writing about cancer, but it may be apt in relation to survivor's guilt. It's difficult to be a survivor if your buddies didn't make it. Survivors often feel more weariness than celebration.

I don't mean to suggest that survivor's guilt is ever-present in the minds of those of us with cancer. It's not. It just flits in and out of our consciousness, especially when another death occurs.

Sometimes it helps just to recognize this guilt and give it a name.

I've often written that cancer brings a profound sense of community. It's really the best thing that came out of my cancer. But by bringing connection, community also brings loss.

I've found that it's also beneficial to memorialize those who have died. Memorials can take the form of donations, participating in cancer walks, volunteering, or simply planting flowers in their honor. Those we have lost would be pleased to know that life continues.

Donating Blood and Organs

In an earlier chapter I wrote about fumbling for words when the Red Cross called and asked if I would donate blood. I had just been diagnosed with cancer and found it hard to say, "I have cancer."

Someone later stopped me and asked, "Well, *can* you give blood after having cancer?"

Good question. I didn't know. I'm also stumped whenever I'm asked if I'm an organ donor. If I check the box, "Yes, I am an organ donor," I worry that whoever gets my kidney will get my breast cancer too.

If I check "No, I am not an organ donor," I feel like I have to justify it by writing, "I'd like to donate, but I've had cancer and you probably wouldn't want my organs anyway." (It's hard to fit all of that on the back of my driver's license.)

It turns out that many people who've had cancer *can* donate both blood and organs.

According to the American Red Cross, being diagnosed with leukemia or lymphoma disqualifies a person from donating, but many others who have had cancer can donate if they have been cancer free for at least one year. Guidelines vary from one blood bank to the next, so call for the specific policies in your area.

An interesting article appeared in the medical journal *Lancet* in May 2007. The researchers identified individuals who had received blood transfusions from people who were later diagnosed with cancer. These donors likely had early cancers that weren't yet detected. The study looked at the recipients of these blood donations and found that they had no greater risk of developing cancer than did the general public.

What about donating kidneys and such after death? I called the United Network for Organ Sharing, the national organization that coordinates organ donations, to see if I can donate my organs. They encourage everyone, even sick people, to be organ donors. Donated organs are given a variety of tests to be sure they are usable. Cancer does not necessarily prevent a person's organs from being used to help someone else. It's the transplant team's job to sort out what they can use and what they can't.

That was a relief. I like checking the box "I am an organ donor."

Survivors Can Help the Newly Diagnosed

People who have had cancer are often asked for advice by those who are newly diagnosed. And quite a few of us feel compelled to give our advice whether it's requested or not.

Some of these conversations are clearly beneficial to the person who's newly diagnosed, while other conversations leave them looking mostly befuddled and/or terrified.

Some general guidelines might be useful:

* The most important piece of advice for the survivor is to do more listening than talking. The conversation isn't about you—it's about the person who was just diagnosed. When someone tells that you that they have just been diagnosed with cancer, they're looking more for understanding than for advice.

✳ The other very important guideline is to make the distinction between sharing your own experiences versus telling the newly diagnosed what's best for them. It's fine to say, "This is what I did," but don't say, "This is what you should do."

✳ People who are newly diagnosed tend to worry about "what if" scenarios. They ask themselves: What if the cancer has spread? What if my treatment doesn't work? What if my spouse breaks an ankle and can't drive the car to buy groceries for our family? These thoughts aren't always rational, but they're understandable. Survivors don't need to make the newly diagnosed feel even more anxious by sharing every bad experience they've ever had or heard about.

✳ Something else to keep in mind during your visit is that you don't need to be irrationally positive, but you shouldn't be aggressively negative either.

✳ Finally, no matter how serious the diagnosis, it's important for the person to maintain hope. Not only hope for a cure, but hope for a smooth treatment process.

In sum, survivors can best help the newly diagnosed by listening and supporting. As the Shaker saying goes, "Let your words be few and seasoned with grace."

Beginning to Talk About Hospice

I often talk with individuals who are receiving treatment for advanced cancer but who are also wondering, at some level, if it's time for hospice. Many tell me that they've made the mental shift to focus on the quality of life rather than the quantity of life, but then add that they haven't contacted hospice or even discussed the possibility because "their family isn't there yet."

It is a difficult topic to discuss and that contributes to the fact that many people receive hospice care only during their final few days rather than their final few months. That's too bad because hospice is much more about living than it is about dying. When I'm ready for hospice, I want to be there long enough to enjoy the entire vacation, not just the final landing.

My advice to people is to contact their local hospice before they need it. I compare it to high school sophomores and juniors beginning to explore colleges. Visiting a college campus does not commit a person to attend that college or even to apply there. It just makes one familiar with the options that are available when the time is right.

Another advantage of contacting hospice early is having the opportunity to discuss those difficult end-of-life issues in the best possible setting. It's so much better to have these discussions *before* there's a crisis. Social workers and other hospice staff members can gently ask the right questions so that the patient's wishes are clear and heard by everyone. Again, this sets nothing in stone, but it does provide a framework for making decisions when they have to be made in the future.

Unlike hospice, which is for the terminally ill (usually defined as having a life expectancy of six months or less), palliative care is available to anyone with a serious illness, without regard to life expectancy or to treatment status (you can still be engaged in curative treatment).

Palliative care is primarily a consultative service that focuses on symptom control and helping individuals and families communicate about end-of-life decisions. This is what the people who work in palliative care do on a daily basis, and they're really good at it.

I also encourage patients to speak openly with their physicians about how long and under which conditions they wish to continue treatment. Other members of the patient's health-care team are also willing to listen and provide guidance.

If you are receiving chemotherapy, you might find it easiest to begin having these conversations with the chemo nurses. (Chemo nurses and their patients love each other. That's just the way it is.) Bringing up the topic is better than OK, it's encouraged.

I personally want to know when hospice is a reasonable option, not when it becomes the only option. The more you communicate, the more you get what you really want.

What to Say When Cancer Returns

I recently gave a talk at a conference for radiation therapists about how to support patients undergoing cancer treatment.

One attendee said, "I know how to help patients when they come in for treatment for the first time. But I stumble over my words when a patient comes back for treatment because they've had a recurrence. What can I say to help them?"

It's a very good question. When cancer returns, the focus usually shifts from curing the cancer to controlling the cancer. It's an entirely different situation from the initial diagnosis, and both the patient and health professional know it.

The patient is likely discouraged because they again have cancer, their prognosis may not be good, and they are facing more treatment that wasn't much fun the first time around.

As evidenced by the question at the conference, even health professionals can feel awkward knowing what to say.

A woman at the conference raised her hand and said, "What I say is that I'm sorry that you've had a recurrence, but we are here for you and we will take good care of you."

It's a simple, honest response that I hope to hear if I ever have a recurrence. The phrase, "I'm sorry," is such a human and caring response.

And "being here for you" and "taking good care of you" are comforting words when comfort is needed more than anything.

When cancer comes back, you know the future is uncertain and you aren't reassured by hearing someone say, "You'll beat this."

You are reassured when your family, friends, and caregivers recognize your reality and are with you for whatever comes.

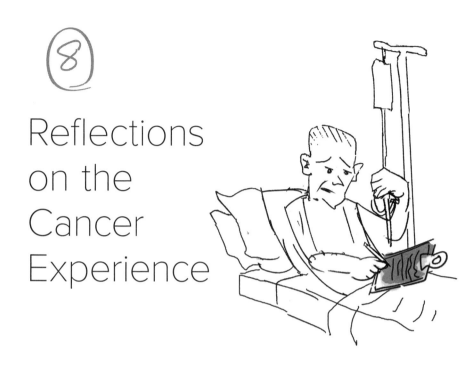

Reflections on the Cancer Experience

Small Acts of Heroism

Heroism in the cancer world—the world I inhabit—isn't the heroism that we see in the movies. It's far more nuanced and, well, real. What I see are daily acts of courage that occur without fanfare but deserve to be noticed.

Simply beginning cancer treatment is a courageous act. Surgery, chemotherapy, and radiation therapy are scary for everyone. I often hear people say afterward, "I never thought I could do it, but I did."

Here are examples of the courage I see:

* There was a young man who decided to quit smoking just as he began chemotherapy. At an age when it's easy

to stick one's head in the sand or blame everyone else, he acknowledged his problems and dealt with them.

* There was the woman who managed to keep working during months of difficult chemotherapy by adapting her work schedule to the rhythms of the treatment.

* There was a man with mental illness who underwent treatment with remarkable dignity and courage.

* There was the guy who hated hospitals and doctors, but came with his wife to support her quietly through every one of her appointments and treatments.

* There were the women who crowded the hospital room of a colleague who was just diagnosed with cancer. No one knew quite what to say, but they knew that being there was important.

* There was the man who stepped in and helped his older brother feel connected and supported during his final months.

* There was the couple that was so loving toward each other and so gracious to everyone else in the chemo suite that they made us all better by just being near.

Time and time again, I see cancer bring out the best in people. Maybe we're at our best when we deal with what's real and cancer certainly is just that. People do their best to get through their treatment, through their illness, or simply through their day. It's the small and seemingly simple acts of courage that constantly amaze and inspire me. We should all take note of the people whose lives have been touched by cancer and recognize the courage they have shown by doing what they thought they could not do.

The Ugly Stepsister of Cancer

There's a warm and fuzzy side to breast cancer. Not the disease itself, which is life-disruptive at its best and deadly at its worst. But there are celebratory races with survivors crossing the finish line with arms raised in triumph, magazine covers honoring celebrities who have survived the disease, and pink ribbons seemingly everywhere.

Other cancers receive less attention. These cancers may not have a warm and fuzzy side, but we agree that people diagnosed with them deserve our support and kindness.

But one cancer is noteworthy for the lack of empathy and compassion it elicits.

"Lung cancer is the ugly stepsister of cancer," was how one person described it to me.

When she was diagnosed, most people assumed that she smoked. She didn't. (Some 10 to 15 percent of people diagnosed with lung cancer are nonsmokers. For reasons not fully understood, lung cancer is more common in nonsmoking women than in nonsmoking men.)

Even her friends who knew she didn't smoke interrogated her to find the cause. There was an underlying sense that if she wasn't at fault, someone or something else was.

Blame seems to be a common theme with lung cancer. People with other cancers aren't blamed. We don't tend to accuse them or even wonder if they did something to cause their cancers. The cancer just is.

Anyone who has had cancer can tell you how difficult it was to get the diagnosis and then to share that news with family and friends. Imagine how much more difficult it would be if you sensed people thinking—or even saying—"Well, that's what you get for smoking."

And, assuming that an individual did smoke, what difference does that make once they have lung cancer? Should we be less compassionate or less supportive? Of course not.

I'm hardly an apologist for smokers or for the tobacco industry. I hate it when smokers foul my air and increase my insurance rates. I make it a point not to enter a business if I see employees smoking near its front door. And I want to shake sense into young people when I see them lighting up.

But if you have lung cancer, you don't need blame. You need kindness and support, given without judgment.

Veterinary Oncology

I had the privilege of meeting recently with a group of veterinary oncologists and technicians at the Cornell University College of Veterinary Medicine.

Veterinary oncologists diagnose and treat cancers in dogs and cats. Just as in humans, cancer care in animals may involve surgery, chemotherapy, and radiation therapy.

What struck me first was that these vets and techs were such nice people. That's a trait they share in common with oncology professionals who work with humans. I think that individuals drawn to oncology tend to be unusually warm-hearted and caring. They have to be because they work with people in the most stressful of situations.

Oncology is also an intellectually challenging field because cancer is so complex. A treatment that works for one individual may not work for another individual with seemingly the exact same cancer.

Oncologists who treat people have to understand different cancers and individual variation, but at least they're dealing with a single species. Oncologists who treat animals have all kinds of tails thumping in their waiting rooms.

The biggest difference, of course, is that treatment decisions are made not by the patient (i.e., the pet), but by the pet owner.

In humans, treatment decisions are so much easier when the patient clearly states his or her wishes. If the patient can't or won't be clear as to what they want, the family generally steps in, but this can be fraught with miscommunication and misunderstandings. Is the decision best for the patient, or for the family? It gets confusing and often stressful.

In the vet world, the pet owner is always the communicator and decision maker. Understanding what your pet wants isn't necessarily obvious. And pet owners can struggle in deciding what's in their own best interests.

Special mention should be made of the vet technicians who work in oncology. In human oncology, patients (and family members) often talk more comfortably and at greater length with the nurses and radiation therapists than with the doctors. The same can be true in veterinary oncology. The techs are often there with the pet owner when the vet leaves the room. They listen, answer questions, and provide an extra dose of kindness when it's most needed.

The financial considerations in vet oncology are more explicit than with humans where cancer treatment is largely covered by insurance. If your dog has cancer, the finances are clear. The vet might say, "Treating your dog's cancer will cost $5,000." Since there's no insurance, that money will come out of your own pocket.

Some owners feel badly that they can't afford the cost and have to forego treatment. Other owners feel guilty spending large sums of money on a pet that wouldn't live many years longer with or without cancer.

If curative treatment is not pursued for whatever reason, veterinary oncologists are also expert in providing palliative care, which—just as in humans—focuses on symptom control and maintaining quality of life.

The most poignant situations are those in which both the pet and the pet owner have cancer. The emotional overtones are everywhere. If the pet dies, is the pet owner next? Or if the owner dies, who will care for the pet?

None of this is simple. It seems that everything we know about cancer is complicated—the disease itself and the emotional entanglements that come with it. I now know that this is as true for veterinary oncologists as it is for human oncologists.

New Nurses and Cancer Patients

Most everyone is uncertain and tentative when first talking with people who are in treatment for cancer. What should you say? What should you not say?

This uncertainty is just as true for health professionals as it is for members of the general public. Even hospital employees sometimes feel tongue-tied when cancer is the diagnosis.

I recently spoke with a class of nursing students at Tompkins Cortland Community College. One woman raised her hand and said, "I'll soon graduate and begin working in a hospital. What should I do to help my patients who have cancer?"

I thought it was a great question, and I've since asked several experienced oncology nurses what they would have shared with the students. This is what they said:

* Don't be afraid of silence. Sometimes you can best support patients by simply being with them without talking.

* Don't reflexively say, "Everything will be fine," or some other reassuring sentiment. It's better to ask, "How are you doing with all of this?"

* Don't assume that what you would want is what the patient should want.

* Be vigilant about pain control. If the patient is in pain, call the doctor. If the patient continues to be in pain, call the doctor again.

* Gently remind patients that they—not their family members or even their doctors—are in charge of treatment decisions.

* Listen to the patients, especially those who have had cancer for a while. They know much more about their cancer than you do.

* Ask patients to tell you their story in their own words. You'll learn about their cancer and about them.

* Be aware of the patient's social situation. Is there support at home? Is the patient likely to fall between the cracks and not receive care after leaving the hospital?

* Use each patient as a learning experience—study the patient's specific type of cancer. What you learn will stay with you because you have a face to go with that diagnosis.

✳ Understand that cancer affects the entire family. Loved ones are often more stressed than the person with cancer.

✳ Be aware of support programs within the hospital (e.g., the chaplain) and in the community (e.g., cancer support organizations) and suggest them to patients when appropriate.

✳ If you have questions, contact the hospital's oncology nurses. They're usually happy to talk about their work and share their knowledge with you.

Several of the nurses I talked with said that they never expected to work in oncology, but they do and they love it. One put it this way, "I once thought cancer was about death and dying, but it's not. It's all about life and living."

The Guys at the Corner Table

Every Friday morning at 8:00 AM, a group of men get together for breakfast at the Royal Court Restaurant in Ithaca. Construction workers, teachers, salesmen, firefighters. Some are retired while others stop by on their way to work. What's noteworthy is that our paths would never have crossed except for our one shared experience—we've all had cancer.

There are several regulars in the group, but newcomers join us almost every week. It's common for people to first join us when they're sorting through their treatment options. The guys at the table don't really give advice, but we do share our personal experiences. And we provide a nonjudgmental forum so people with decisions to make can freely discuss what they've been considering. They sort of test-drive their thinking at our table. (Sometimes it's easier to bounce around ideas with people who aren't members of your own family).

And there are times when we talk mostly about things other than cancer. Sports, politics, business, and other topics pop up almost every week.

It's interesting that so many types of cancers are represented: prostate, colon, lung, melanoma, bladder, breast, lymphoma, leukemia. The differences between our cancers are far less important than their commonalities. We've all learned to live with uncertainty.

No wonder that some military veterans in the group say that the bond we form is very similar to the bond that they formed with their buddies in the service. People connect quickly and deeply when life and death are daily realities.

I routinely talk with community groups, and I'm sometimes asked if anything good emerged from my having cancer. I used to respond that having cancer forced me to reexamine my priorities in life and to focus on what's truly important. I still value that, but I'm beginning to realize that the greatest good that emerged from my cancer is a strong sense of community.

Cancer brings me in contact with people I wouldn't have met in any other way. It's the ultimate equalizer: We're all looking to connect with others who understand.

I'm constantly reminded of this when we get together on Friday mornings. When we leave, some guys are heading off for a little fishing while others might be going to the hospital for a CT scan. But everyone has shared a connection—and a good breakfast—with old and new friends at the corner table.

Cancer and the Nature of Hope

Cancer and hope are two topics that often intersect.

People with cancer sometimes wonder if maintaining hope in the face of a grim diagnosis is a good idea or a bad idea.

My response is that hope is always good, but it's a mistake to define hope strictly in the context of being cured.

When a person is first diagnosed with cancer, hope and cure do overlap. People hope that they will be cured. Even if the survival rate for your type of cancer is only 10 percent, somebody has to be in that 10 percent, and it might as well be you.

Or it might be said, "People with your cancer can expect to live about twelve months." What that means is that half of the people with your cancer will live longer than twelve months.

Statistics provide guideposts, but they don't dictate what will happen to a specific individual.

Of course, cancer can metastasize or otherwise advance to the point that a cure is unrealistic.

But does this mean giving up hope? No, not at all. But it does mean reframing your concept of hope to something other than a cure.

Many people who can't be cured can hope for months or years of continuing to live with a good quality of life.

Even people with a terminal diagnosis can and should have hope. The hope may be as modest as having a good weekend or as significant as a reconciliation with an estranged family member.

Hope is somehow at the core of our being human, even when one's current situation is difficult.

And there is the hope that our lives have had and will continue to have meaning.

The Good That Emerged

A friend with cancer wrote me to say how she now experiences moments of intense appreciation.

Just walking her dog at Buttermilk State Park filled her with tears. Not tears of sadness, but tears of unabashed appreciation of that gorgeous moment.

The dog, the forest, the beauty. They made her cry.

She said that she never had such intense feelings before her cancer.

Her comments got me to thinking that good often emerges from serious illness.

I asked attendees at a recent cancer support group if anything positive came out of their disease. Each person said yes.

One woman waved her hand around the table and said that she found a remarkable sense of community with others who also have cancer. "We're in the same boat—we understand each other." She added softly, "I love that."

Another person said that cancer builds community because it's a great equalizer. "It doesn't matter if you're black or white, rich or poor, man or woman. We're all sick and we're all scared. I don't know the name of the person who's getting chemo in the chair next to me, but he's like a brother to me now."

Other people at the support group saw cancer as a personal challenge. One guy said, "Cancer is the scariest thing I've ever faced. But I found that I had the strength to get through it. I didn't think I could, but I did and I'm proud of that."

Nearly everyone expressed gratitude that they no longer take anything for granted. "I give thanks every day," said a woman, accompanied by nods from all around the table.

Trust and faith were two recurring themes in the group. So much about cancer is uncertain that one has to plunge forward even though no one knows for certain what will happen. "Trust is hard for me, but I had to trust my doctors," said one man. "And once I gave that trust, I began to relax a little."

Many also described a renewed sense of spirituality when confronted with cancer. Faith often provides comfort during our most difficult times.

I'm so often impressed by how people respond to cancer with dignity, strength, and grace. Cancer isn't good and I wouldn't wish it on anyone. But only a person touched by serious illness could have written, "I was suddenly overwhelmed at how lucky I was to be alive; I was experiencing this sunny day in the forest with my beloved puppy and I started crying because it was so gorgeous."

New Year's Wishes

New Year's wishes take on added urgency and poignancy when you or a loved one has cancer. These are my wishes for everyone affected by cancer:

I wish that everyone with cancer had a kind, steady, and supportive companion beside them.

I wish that everyone with cancer who has a kind, steady, and supportive companion beside them recognizes and appreciates the treasure that they have.

I wish that people with cancer were immune to other diseases and misfortunes. We should only have to deal with one bad thing at a time.

I wish that bake sales, community barbeques, and other events to raise money for individuals with cancer weren't necessary.

I wish that people with cancer weren't beaten over the head with the importance of positive thinking.

I wish that people didn't feel awkward talking about rectal and anal cancers.

I wish that people received hospice care for many weeks—not just days—before their deaths.

I wish that more people recognized that reducing one's own risk of cancer isn't confusing or dependent on expensive supplements. Just try to maintain a good weight, exercise, eat a balanced and largely plant-based diet, and don't smoke.

I wish that people understood that we can help prevent cancers in our children and grandchildren by taking better care of our environment.

I wish that the relatives, friends, and neighbors of people newly diagnosed with cancer refrained from giving advice (except when requested).

I wish that kindness was consistently recognized and valued as an essential component of cancer treatment and care.

I wish that every cancer patient understood that reality and hope aren't mutually exclusive.

Supporting Others with Cancer

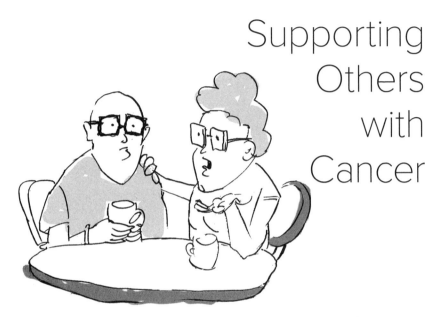

Helping Friends with Cancer

Nearly everyone has had a friend, neighbor, coworker, or acquaintance diagnosed with cancer. Most people want to be helpful, but may fear being intrusive or simply getting in the way of the immediate family. In general, what those of us with cancer most appreciate from our friends are help with practical matters and the maintenance, as much as possible, of a sense of being normal.

Here are a few suggestions for what you should and shouldn't do:

Do

* Send cards of support and encouragement (e-mail just isn't the same).

* Walk their dogs, cut their grass, or shovel their walk.

* Offer to bring mutual friends over to watch a sporting event or other favorite TV show.

* Offer to watch their kids for an evening or weekend.

* Drop off meals that can be frozen.

* Take their trash cans to the curb.

* Offer to drive them to appointments.

* Offer to organize other friends who may want to help by cooking or driving.

* Send small gifts.

* Send another card.

* Take the initiative for staying in touch. The person with cancer is often short of both time and energy.

* Extend small kindnesses.

* Make a donation in their honor to an organization they value.

Don't

* Provide unsolicited advice about how they should treat their cancer.

* Assume that your friend is a different person because they've been diagnosed with cancer.

* Be afraid of talking about normal stuff. People with cancer usually enjoy taking a break from cancer.

* Stay too long when visiting. If the patient is looking tired, let them rest.

* Ask, "How can I help?" That puts the burden on the patient to think of things. It's better to call and offer something concrete such as, "I'm heading to the grocery store this afternoon. Can I pick up something for you?"

* Be nosy. It's fine to ask how the person is doing, but don't pry for details. If they want to tell you, they will.

A person who recently went through cancer treatment told me that the friends he valued the most were those who found the "sweet spot." That is, they acknowledged his cancer but still treated him like he was still the same person. It's a balancing act that may take some fine-tuning and practice, but it's worth the effort.

What to Say—and Not Say

Most people find it awkward when first talking with a friend or acquaintance who has just been diagnosed with cancer. Even though nearly everyone is well-intentioned, many say things that hurt or mystify more than they comfort.

Based on my own experiences as a cancer patient and my conversations with others with cancer, here are some suggestions for what you should and shouldn't say:

What not to say:

Don't worry. You'll be fine. Everyone's natural instinct is to reassure the newly diagnosed that everything will be

OK. While encouraging words are welcome, most people just diagnosed with cancer will be worried. Rather than dismissing those worries, acknowledge them.

That's too bad about your cancer, but I could be hit by a bus tomorrow. No one in the history of civilization has ever found comfort in these words, but people say it all the time.

Do you smoke? People with lung cancer get asked this routinely. This is blaming, not supporting. People seem to ask this question for their own peace of mind. "You smoked and got lung cancer. I don't smoke, therefore I don't have to worry."

You have to see this doctor or have this treatment or begin this cancer-fighting diet. If people want your advice, they'll ask for it.

Tell me how I can help. This comment often comes from the heart, but it puts the burden on the person with cancer to think of and assign tasks. It's far better just to do things.

What to say:

I'm so sorry. This is a good and honest response.

How are you doing with all of this? A simple question like this lets the person with cancer take the lead and opens the door for conversation.

Would you like to grab a cup of coffee and talk?

I'm keeping you in my thoughts and prayers. Positive energy always helps, in whatever form works for you and the person with cancer.

One friend describes two layers of response whenever she tells someone that she has cancer. The first layer is immediate, honest, and from the gut: "Oh no. I'm so sorry." The second layer is when the person begins saying those things they *think* they should say: "You'll be fine. You'll be playing tennis in a month." She wishes that people would stop talking after the "I'm so sorry."

As with other difficult conversations, the specific words are less important than the tangible presence of friends and loved ones. It's OK if the words get a bit tangled—it's the heart that matters.

Advocating for a Loved One

It's extremely helpful for a person with cancer to have an advocate present during doctor's appointments and hospital stays.

The most important role for the advocate is to understand and be supportive of the patient and the patient's wishes.

Above all, a good advocate needs to be a good listener. Listen to the patient. And listen to the health professionals.

Most problems occur when loved ones confuse their own wishes and agenda with those of the patient. This isn't done maliciously. More often, it's based on assumptions of what's best for the patient without actually asking the patient.

It's entirely normal for loved ones to have their own agendas. But understand that the patient's agenda and their loved ones' agendas aren't necessarily one and the same.

It can be helpful for patients and their loved ones to separately write down their wishes and priorities. Afterward, compare the lists to see where they overlap and where they differ. This provides clarity and also a springboard for discussion.

Ultimately, though, advocates need to realize that it is the patient and the patient's wishes that take precedence. Here are a few additional suggestions for advocates:

* Talk with the patient before appointments to write down questions the patient wants to ask.

* Let the patient speak for him or herself.

* Take notes.

* Let the health-care team do its work.

* Report changes in the patient's status to the health professionals, especially ones that aren't obvious. For example, "Sarah seems to have much less energy than she did last month."

* Understand the reality of the situation and maintain reasonable expectations.

* Be a bridge-builder. Connect with providers, other patients, and family members.

* Think of ways to help with nonmedical issues; e.g., household chores that free up the patient's time and energy.

Some people don't think of themselves as advocates because they aren't loud and pushy. In fact, the best advocates are quiet forces who support mostly by their steadfast presence. I heard one patient refer to his advocate as his "designated listener." What a perfect description. We should all have designated listeners.

How to Be a "Groundhog Friend"

I'm often asked how to be a friend to someone with cancer.

I generally answer this question by encouraging them to be good listeners and to be present for their friend in every sense of the word.

The best friends are what I describe as "groundhog friends."

Remember the movie *Groundhog Day* with Bill Murray? The same day kept reappearing. That isn't a good trait for one's day, but it's a terrific trait for a friend of someone with cancer.

When someone is first diagnosed, many people call, send notes, and help in a variety of ways. That's great and those kindnesses are appreciated.

But cancer is more a marathon than a sprint. The challenging time is when the initial outpouring of support slows and the patient still has four months of chemotherapy looming ahead.

A groundhog friend checks on the patient throughout the course of his or her treatment.

A groundhog friend keeps sending notes of support.

A groundhog friend keeps popping up to do things that make the patient's life easier.

A groundhog friend isn't offended by the patient's crankiness on those inevitable bad days.

A groundhog friend doesn't change the subject when the patient has bad news to share.

A groundhog friend keeps filling the patient's freezer with food.

A groundhog friend brings in other friends when the patient is in the mood and keeps them away when he or she isn't.

Above all, a groundhog friend keeps reappearing, day after day.

A Better Phrase than Staying Strong

If your loved one has cancer, you may sense an obligation to be strong. The phrase "Be strong" is branded into our brains, but I wish we had a better phrase to capture the role of the people closest to those with cancer.

Being strong makes me think of Clint Eastwood characters. Never flinching, always moving forward, threatening to beat cancer to a pulp. I, for one, would not be comforted by having Dirty Harry in my chemotherapy room.

Strong sometimes gets confused with stoic. A man in treatment once told me, "My wife tries to be strong and not cry in front of me, but we both know it's an act. We've been married for 45 years and she always cries. It's just who she is. I wish she would cry with me now."

When everyone else goes home, the patient needs someone to stay behind and share his or her reality. With cancer, the reality is sometimes good, sometimes bad, and often uncertain.

I think a better phrase than "being strong" is "being connected." That's what a person with cancer most needs—the sense that a loved one will be there and be connected for whatever comes.

One critical role for the loved one is to focus on the patient's quality of life: Is treatment affecting the patient's ability to sleep? To eat? Are they experiencing pain? Sometimes doctors—and even patients—need to be reminded about the seemingly small things that can make a huge difference in how the person feels. I recently heard one person describe his spouse as his "quality-of-life advocate." He went on to say that everyone needs a quality of life advocate during cancer treatment. I couldn't agree more.

The Challenge of Being a Caretaker

A cancer diagnosis changes the life of the patient and the lives of the people who love the patient. It can be especially challenging for loved ones because they may want to appear strong and optimistic even though they're scared to death on the inside.

In addition to worrying about *their* loved one's cancer, they may be running the household, struggling with piles of incomprehensible insurance forms, communicating with far-flung family members, and trying to earn enough money to pay the mounting bills. Life doesn't get much more stressful.

I talk with many people who acknowledge this stress, but who also say that helping their loved one through cancer was the best thing they ever did.

What's essential is to understand that the role of the loved one is to support and comfort, not to "fix" the problem. Men tend to have a harder time with this because we somehow expect ourselves to fix whatever is broken. Cancer isn't always fixable.

When people are diagnosed with cancer, they don't want their loved ones to say, "I promise you that you'll be cured." Nobody can guarantee that. Further, that kind of statement tends to cut off more honest dialogue.

What they want to hear is, "I love you and I'll be here with you for whatever comes."

It's OK to be scared and share that with one another. That's real.

That's one thing about cancer—it's all too real. There's no getting around the fact that it's a bad disease and that there are many unknowns. Sharing that reality will make it more manageable for both of you.

There are things that people who have a loved one with cancer can do for their own well-being:

* Carve out some time for yourself, even a few minutes each day. Exercise is especially beneficial because it burns off tension, improves your sleep, and recharges your body.

* Create an outlet where you can talk about you on a regular basis. Therapists, pastors, and long-time friends are good sources of support. Don't try to do everything yourself. Accept offers of help.

There's no way to make caring for a seriously ill loved one easy or painless. It can be exhausting at best and absolutely harrowing at worst. But for many of us, it's the single most courageous and important act of our lives.

Helping from a Distance

I once received a letter from a man serving time in prison asking how he could help his mother who was ill with cancer.

As I wrote back to offer suggestions, I recall thinking that this was an extreme example of long-distance caregiving. He literally couldn't visit his mother and his ability to communicate with her was limited.

There are countless other situations in which someone wants to help a loved one with cancer, but geography makes it impossible to pop over with a bowl of soup and a hug.

But there are ways to help and support, even if you can't be there in person:

* Send notes of support. Let them know that you're sending positive thoughts.

* Realize that people with cancer often receive lots of cards when they are first diagnosed. The cards that they receive weeks and months later—when they're tired of cancer and its treatment—are especially treasured.

* Don't be discouraged if you don't receive a response. People in the middle of treatment often need to conserve their energy. I've known people to respond seemingly out of the blue years later to say how much those cards meant.

* Educate yourself about their cancer. Colon cancer is very different from thyroid cancer. Acquiring a basic knowledge will help you understand what they're going through and facilitate communication.

* Call, even if it feels awkward at first. It's OK to say simply, "I'm sorry you have cancer." People don't usually remember what you said, but they'll remember that you called. And don't worry about waking someone up or disturbing them. They more than likely have an answering machine.

* Small gifts, unrelated to illness, are always welcome.

* Reach out to the primary caregiver. They may need an outlet or simply a recognition of their difficult role.

* I've had friends take part in cancer walks and raise money in my honor. I love when that happens.

* If writing or calling is difficult, you can always send good and positive thoughts. As one friend with cancer told me, "Prayers, good vibes, thinking of me—I'll take it in any form."

More than anything, the person with cancer will appreciate the sense of staying connected with you and staying connected with his or her "normal" life. Cancer tends to throw everything into upheaval. Distant friends and family can help people with cancer maintain their sense of who they were before cancer and, hopefully, the life to which they will return when treatment ends.

Helping Those We Don't Like

I often suggest practical ways to help people with cancer. Giving support to nice people is relatively easy. You *want* to bring them soup and give them a hug.

But contrary to what you see in the movies, not everyone with cancer is angelic. Some of us are cranky. Others are downright unpleasant.

Whether one likes them or not, unpleasant people need support, too.

In my experience, unpleasant people with cancer were unpleasant people before they had cancer. And nothing about cancer is going to make them any happier.

The first unpleasant person who comes to your mind might be a member of your family. Perhaps it's a parent or a sibling. Or it could be a neighbor, member of your faith community, or coworker.

If this unpleasant person gets cancer, you may feel some obligation to help. This sense of obligation might be heightened if the person is socially isolated which, not surprisingly, tends to happen to unpleasant people.

So what to do?

My suggestion is to reach out to them by calling, visiting, and offering to take them to appointments. But don't expect them to smile, be gracious, or appreciate your assistance.

We're taught by Hollywood that cranky people have hearts of gold and twinkles in their eyes. I've known several people like that, but I've also known people who seem to have hearts of stone, and the word "twinkle" will never, ever be used to describe them.

But that doesn't mean that we can't help in one way or another, even if it's a small gesture and we have to force a smile.

A friend of mine, referring to her sister, put it to me this way, "I don't like her, but I'm here for her."

There's a lot of wisdom and love in that statement. Sometimes we help simply because it's the right thing to do.

If Your Mom or Dad Has Cancer

I sometimes hear from middle-aged friends who tell me that their mother or father was just diagnosed with cancer. They then launch into their plans for their parent's treatment: "I think Mom should...."

This is when I ask, "What does your mom want?"

This question is usually met by a four- or five-second pause, followed by a hesitant, "What do you mean?"

"I mean, what does your mom want? Have you asked her?" You'd be surprised how often Mom hasn't been asked.

In some cases, adult children want Mom to have the most aggressive treatment possible, even if that treatment is likely to extend her life for only a few months and at the cost of making her miserable.

In other cases, children want to take their mother across the country to the world's expert on her disease when she would be more comfortable staying with the doctors who know her and have treated her for many years.

Sometimes the most aggressive therapy is the best approach, and sometimes it does make sense to travel to see the world's expert. But, please, don't make assumptions about what your mother or father wants. Ask.

It's often helpful to involve your parent's primary-care physician in the decision-making process. The specialists involved in your parent's care will focus on what can be done. The primary-care physician can help your mother or father sort through what should be done, based on your parent's overall condition, personal wishes, and a host of other factors.

What's most important for a daughter or son in dealing with a parent's cancer is simply to be present for your mother or father. Be available when your parent wants to talk and supportive of the choices she makes. This is hard for many of us because we're accustomed to fixing things. We tend to focus too much on the fix and not enough on the person.

Health-care providers will naturally focus on your parent's cancer. As a family member, you have the opportunity and privilege of focusing on your mother or father as a person. It's the best gift you'll ever give your parent.

Understanding Friends with Cancer

I recently had a conversation with a woman whose good friend was diagnosed with cancer. She hoped that the cancer wouldn't change their friendship, but it did. The change, though, was temporary. As she told me, "My friend had to go through a process to come to terms with her cancer—I just didn't understand that at first."

When people are diagnosed with a life-threatening illness, they aren't sure what they should think, and they're even less sure what they should say to family and friends. It's a period of emotional churning more than of clear insight. Most people need time to sort things out in their own minds before discussing them with anyone outside of their immediate families.

But friends often want to know some of the specifics of the patient's condition and the proposed treatment. Imagine having a long-time friend that you've shared everything with. All of sudden, she has cancer and she's not talking. It's easy to feel left out.

As this person told me, "I wondered if she was telling other people about her cancer but not me. I felt out of the loop."

Several weeks later, though, this person realized that, "This has to be about her, not about me." She was feeling left out because she was focusing on her own needs and not on the needs of the person with cancer. Once this realization hit, she was able to relax and let her friend's internal process take its natural course.

She decided to be a silent friend, to listen, to be available, to be supportive, but not to pry. She left flowers on her doorstop, sent cards, and remained a steady presence. In turn, her friend called on her more and more because she knew that she wouldn't get questions that she didn't want to answer.

This is how Rachel Naomi Remen, author of the wonderful books *Kitchen Table Wisdom* and *My Grandfather's Blessings*, described this gift of listening: "The most basic and powerful way to connect to another person is to listen. Just listen. Perhaps the most important thing we ever give each other is our attention.… A loving silence often has far more power to heal and to connect than the most well-intentioned words."

And gentle silence often leads to honest conversations when the time is right. When the woman's friend with cancer was ready to talk, the floodgates opened wide.

There was so much that her friend had to say, but it just wasn't time until that particular moment.

Cancer can and does change friendships, but the best friendships are resilient and will re-emerge after a period of adjustment. To be a true friend is to respect the privacy, process, and timetable of the person with cancer. When in doubt, just listen with an open heart.

Being Present

Being diagnosed with cancer is like entering a dark and unfamiliar place. Imagine being suddenly transported deep inside a cave. You sense creepy things all around and it's hard to see the path that may lead you out. It's disorienting and scary.

This metaphor was suggested to me by Reverend Tim Dean of Cayuga Medical Center's Department of Spiritual Care. He went on to describe the role of a hospital chaplain as that of being present with people when they're in these dark places.

Darkness is a good metaphor for the uncertainty that accompanies cancer. I didn't fully appreciate this until I was diagnosed with the disease. The cause of the cancer was unknown, more than one treatment was possible, and my future was less than guaranteed. We all live with uncertainty, but with cancer, that uncertainty is palpable.

At the Cancer Resource Center, we train new volunteers to provide assistance to those affected by cancer. The volunteers are taught to listen, provide emotional support, and identify resources. Most of all, our volunteers and staff provide a sense of presence. That is, we're there with people when their world seems so uncertain.

All of us—not just chaplains and cancer center volunteers—have the ability to be present with friends and family who are dealing with a cancer diagnosis. Too often, loved ones assume that their most important role is to fix the problem. It's not. Their more important role is to be there beside the person with cancer.

It's possible to be present even if you live elsewhere. I recently talked with a woman whose best friend sent her a daily e-mail of support during her months of treatment. Those messages meant so much to her that she hand-copied each one into a notebook. She cried when she showed that notebook to me.

That kind of friend adds light to the darkness and makes it a less scary place.

Visiting Those in the Hospital

People with cancer are sometimes hospitalized, and their friends often want to visit to offer support and encouragement. Understanding some general guidelines will help make the visit a positive experience for everyone:

* Keep the visits brief. People in the hospital are generally quite ill and have limited energy. If you stay long, it puts a burden on them to keep you entertained. Visits of ten to fifteen minutes are often best.

* Be sure that the patient wants visitors. Call ahead to see if visiting is a good idea and, if so, what time of day is preferred.

* If a visit isn't possible, send a card. And bring a card with you if you do visit. Patients often put those cards on the wall and feel comforted by them.

* Don't visit if you're sick. The last thing a hospitalized patient needs is your germs.

* Wash your hands before entering the room, even if you're healthy. There are sinks and alcohol-based hand cleansers throughout the hospital. Use them.

* Don't wear strong fragrances. Some ill patients are acutely sensitive to scents. And please don't smoke before visiting—the smell lingers on your clothes.

* If doctors or other health professionals enter the room, excuse yourself and go into the hallway unless the patient specifically asks that you stay.

❋ If family members are present, realize that the patient needs private time with them. Give your regards, but don't linger in the room.

❋ Don't sit on the patient's bed unless you are asked to do so. Patients are often physically uncomfortable and they don't want to be jostled or cramped.

❋ Don't hug the patient unless it's clear that they want that hug. If you've just had surgery, a hug can be painful.

❋ Don't whine about things in your life. No one wants to hear, "I'm sorry that you have lung cancer, Joe, but I just got a parking ticket and I'm really steamed."

❋ Don't pry into the patient's health. If they want to share with you, they'll share with you. It's fine to ask how they're feeling, but leave it at that.

❋ Don't be afraid of silence. Sometimes it's the best support you can provide.

As is so often the case, what's in your heart is more important than the words you say. When people are seriously ill, they sense kindness and support around them. Your visits, cards, prayers, and positive thoughts do make a difference.

Holiday Gifts

I have been thinking about gift suggestions for people who are being treated for cancer and for those who have recently completed treatment.

As a starting point, my recommendation is to give gifts of life rather than gifts of cancer. No matter how well-intentioned the gift, I become cranky if I find my Christmas stocking stuffed with pink ribbons or books with titles like, *Cancer Is a Special Blessing* or *I Beat Cancer with an Eggplant Diet.*

Give people an opportunity to think about something other than cancer.

In addition to everything else, cancer is expensive, and disposable money is often tight. Give little luxuries. A gift certificate to a favorite restaurant or to a local theater can be a real treat. Join together with friends and give a person a day of pampering at a local spa.

For the person who's completed treatment, consider something with a future orientation. The time immediately following treatment is often unexpectedly difficult, so help them look ahead. Perhaps tickets to a play that's coming to town in a few months or an upcoming sporting event.

But what if your loved one has advanced cancer and this holiday season may be their last? Gifts with a future orientation might be well intentioned, but they ignore reality.

If a person you love is nearing the end of her life, why not celebrate that life?

A photo album or scrapbook that captures your mother's life will have more meaning for her than a new pair of slippers. Ask her friends and other family members to contribute photos and mementoes. They'll be delighted.

And I think it's a wonderful tribute to make donations in a person's honor *before* they die. Suggest donations to your dad's favorite charity, perhaps creating a special fund in his honor.

Some people say that gifts that celebrate a person's life are wrong because they imply the person is dying.

Hello? If your mom is dying, she knows that she's dying. Giving her a family scrapbook isn't going to push her over the edge.

Holidays bring families together and most of us make special efforts to join loved ones if a family member is seriously ill. Sharing stories is not an admission of impending death—it's a celebration of life and a recognition that a person's life continues to have meaning.

There's no question that holidays take on an added poignancy when a loved one is nearing the end of life. Expect some tears. But expect laughter as well. It's all about life.

Thoughts and Prayer Tree

There's a small tree in the living room of Gary and Mary Ellen Stewart's house in Ithaca, New York. It's covered with cards, letters, and drawings.

At first, a visitor isn't quite sure what it is. It looks somewhat like a Christmas tree, but it's the wrong time of year.

A closer look reveals that everything attached to the tree is offering some form of encouragement. "We're thinking of you." "I'm with you." "I love you."

Gary had the idea of creating this "Thoughts and Prayer Tree" to support Mary Ellen who's nearing the end of chemotherapy. Anyone who has been through chemo—or any cancer treatment—can tell you it's a grueling experience that depletes one's spirits and energy.

Friends and family kept asking Gary how they could help Mary Ellen. He suggested that everyone send cards, letters, and other expressions of support. These soon began arriving and Gary used twist-ties to attach them to a small, artificial

Christmas tree. Gary then took a photo of the tree and sent it out by e-mail, which generated many more cards and letters that were then added.

I tend to stack cards in a pile on the coffee table and leave them there for six weeks when I guiltily stick them into the recycling bin. The Thoughts and Prayer Tree, however, lets these cards and letter become living, three-dimensional expressions of support to be read and savored by everyone in the room.

Mary Ellen told me that the cards and letters were personal and deeply felt, unlike Christmas cards, which often feel mass produced. She was especially touched by cards from people who were dealing with their own illnesses and challenges, but still took the time to reach out and connect with her.

Another special group of cards, often handmade, were from children who would often stop by the Stewart house to visit the tree. They were always so pleased to see their handiwork displayed.

Gary remarked that it's such a good lesson for children, including their 13-year-old son, Ben, who can see how people can and do support one another through difficult times.

I love the idea of a Thoughts and Prayer Tree. It's both simple and powerful.

It also highlights an important lesson. So often we think of someone or pray for someone who's ill or otherwise in need of our support. But we don't always take the time to actually tell them that we're thinking of them or praying for them. We should.

As I was leaving their home, Mary Ellen gazed up at the tree and said, "I never get tired of looking at it."

Mental Illness and Cancer

If anyone deserves a guaranteed place in heaven, it's people who support a loved one who has both serious mental illness and cancer.

This is more common than one might expect. I know of several individuals who are helping family members through cancer after helping them through mental illness for years or even decades.

I've found that many people with mental illness—especially those with a supportive family member—get through cancer treatment remarkably well, sometimes even better than people without mental illness.

Several oncology nurses I've talked with have observed the same thing. One suggested that people with mental illness have developed good coping mechanisms because they've already faced so many challenges in life. Cancer is just one more challenge to add to that list.

I suspect people with mental illness feel some relief that cancer is so tangible. Unlike mental illness—which often exists in shades of gray—cancer tends to be black and white. It shows up in X rays and lab tests. Everyone can see it.

And people with mental illness often develop an almost instinctive sense of which health professionals are trustworthy. If you've been seeing doctors and therapists for years, you get a good sense of who really cares and who is just going through the motions. Oncology nurses and radiation therapists are especially good at creating nurturing and trusting relationships with patients going through cancer treatment.

But few things are as helpful to those with cancer—whether mental illness is involved or not—as having a loved one beside them to provide day-to-day support and practical assistance.

Family relationships are often strained by mental illness, so it's common for the person with mental illness to be isolated. Loved ones who have stayed connected and supportive of those with mental illness have likely worked hard to maintain those relationships.

These family members often ask me how they can help now that their loved one has cancer in addition to mental illness. What I tell them is that their presence and concern count more than anything.

Many of us have already or will receive a diagnosis of cancer *or* mental illness. It's a huge challenge and often life changing. Now imagine dealing with cancer and mental illness at the same time. Many people do so with remarkable courage and grace. I admire them, and I admire their family members who stand near and love them every step of the way.

When Loved Ones Complete Treatment

Most people realize that their loved ones with cancer need special attention when they are beginning treatment.

Fewer people realize that their loved ones also need special attention when they are *finishing* cancer treatment.

Family members generally look forward to the end of treatment because it means that life may get back to normal. They've probably put their own lives on hold for months, and they're eager for a vacation from the whole cancer experience.

People with cancer often have mixed feelings as treatment ends. While they're happy to be rid of the unpleasant side effects of chemotherapy and radiation, they wonder what the future holds. Have they been cured, or will the cancer return?

These fears fade with time, but the months immediately following treatment are especially difficult. Patients miss the security provided by their chemo nurses and radiation therapists. These professionals provided a ready outlet for their questions and fears.

When treatment is over, many patients think about cancer nearly all of the time. They stew over things and they want to talk. The people most likely to be within earshot are loved ones who may be less than enthused about talking about cancer, cancer, and more cancer.

So, how can loved ones help while maintaining their own sanity?

I recommend that they encourage the patient to talk about his or her feelings, but mostly with someone *other* than a loved one. This is a perfect time to join a support group. I joined a group when I found myself in a post-treatment funk and that group provided just the outlet I needed.

In addition to face-to-face groups, there are online discussion groups for nearly every type of cancer and situation. Some people, of course, just don't like groups, and I encourage them to connect on an individual basis with a therapist, pastor, or other professional who can offer emotional support. This can provide some much-needed breathing space for everyone.

Loved ones can also help by gently shifting the focus from illness to wellness. I always caution against making major lifestyle changes *during* cancer treatment, but lifestyle changes *after* treatment often help physically and provide one with a sense of control. And nearly everyone can benefit from a better diet, moderate exercise, and other healthy behaviors.

Stepping Up for Neighbors

As I've mentioned, not everyone with cancer has built-in support. Perhaps the individual has no family, or an event in the past may have caused the family to become estranged. Some people are just loners by nature and have happily kept to themselves through the years. Others are isolated because of mental illness. And some people have burned every bridge that once brought them connection.

I'd like to recognize a small group of people who step up to support a neighbor, a community member, or an acquaintance who would otherwise go through cancer alone.

This support takes many forms. Sometimes it's driving the person to treatment, bringing over a bowl of soup, or helping sort through the stack of bills on the kitchen table. Often, the most important role is to listen as the person comes to grips with having a life-threatening illness.

But I have also seen this support evolve such that the neighbor is the one who helps the patient navigate their final months of life. The neighbor becomes the de facto family—making sure that the patient is loved and that their wishes are carried out. I've even seen neighbors arrange funerals and scatter the individual's ashes afterward.

I don't think we have a word for all of this, but I wish we did. "Saintly" doesn't really work because not all of these caregivers are, well, saintly. More often, they're just normal folk who go to work, drink beer on the weekend, and try to do what's right.

They don't consciously decide to help their neighbor through their final days—it just happens. I suspect they sometimes think, "I really don't want to do this."

But they do.

I often wonder how and why people are able to help their neighbors in this way. It's certainly not done for the recognition or for money. I do believe that most people want to find meaning in life. Helping someone through illness and death—especially someone you have no obligation to help— has to be one of life's most meaningful experiences.

And, as we get older and wiser, many realize that helping a neighbor is how we best save the world.

By the very nature of what they do, these good neighbors are the last ones to leave the funeral home. There's no one left behind to thank them.

If one of you is reading this, know that I thank you. And know that your community is a better place because of you.

Doing What I Do

I often talk with people while they're receiving chemotherapy. Recently, one woman asked, "How long have you been doing this?"

I knew that she was talking about my work at the Cancer Resource Center of the Finger Lakes, so I replied that I've been visiting with cancer patients for more than ten years. She then asked, "How do you do it?"

She went on, "You deal with cancer every single day. Some patients won't ever get better. And nearly everyone you talk with must be scared, sick, or both. Doesn't it depress the hell out of you?"

I've been reflecting on this question ever since.

Although the question was directed to me, it just as easily could have been directed to the doctors, nurses, radiation therapists, and others who work with cancer patients on a regular basis.

I posed the question to a nurse who responded, "Everyone who begins cancer treatment will have an outcome. Sometimes that outcome is a cure, sometimes it's not a cure but a longer life, and sometimes the outcome is that the person dies no matter what we do."

She said, "I can't focus on the outcomes—I focus on the journey. I can make the journey better for people, and doing so brings me satisfaction."

One physician told me she wishes that no one would ever say the words, "There's nothing we can do." She said, "There's always something we can do. We can control pain, we can provide comfort, we can listen."

A hospital chaplain told me that his job is to be with people when they're in dark and scary places. It's not a matter of fixing things. It's a matter of sharing the experience so that no one is alone.

There's an underlying theme to all of these comments. Working with people with cancer requires a focus on what you can do, rather than on what you cannot do. That's why I love this job.

Good News in Cancer

A woman recently stopped me to say that my newspaper columns about cancer were depressing and I should try hard to be more upbeat.

I replied that a column written about cancer has to include some sadness and pain if it's going to be honest.

But I decided to challenge myself and write only positive thoughts, at least this once:

* Health professionals who work regularly with cancer patients are some of the best and most caring people you'll ever meet.

* In general, people are now comfortable talking openly about having cancer. I can't imagine going through cancer and keeping it a secret (which used to be quite common).

* The horrific nausea that was once associated with chemotherapy is now quite rare.

* Cancer support groups provide an amazing opportunity to connect with people from all walks of life. Individuals find community in these groups.

* Some cancers (e.g., testicular) are now curable even at an advanced stage.

* Surgical techniques are far more refined with more attention to cosmetic results. Some cancer surgeries that were once disfiguring (e.g., neck dissections) are now hardly noticeable.

* Radiation therapy is dramatically more sophisticated and precise than it used to be.

* Many of the newest drugs target the underlying biology of the tumor, meaning that treatments are both more effective and less toxic.

* Lung cancer rates are declining because people are smoking less.

* People are often able to live with advanced cancer for many years with a surprisingly good quality of life.

* Our ability to take images inside the body with CT scans, MRIs, and PET scans have reduced the number of surgeries that were once needed to "take a look around."

* I know so many wonderful people who, in one way or another, I've met because of cancer.

I've come to realize that writing about cancer is writing about life. There is progress and pain, and there are many paths to follow with no single path being right for everyone.

Your path through cancer is *your* path to choose.

Resources

Informational Websites

www.medlineplus.gov

A terrific starting point is *Medline Plus*, which is the public online resource of the National Institutes of Health. Visit the website for information on specific types of cancer or other topics (e.g., chemotherapy). A variety of credible sources, thoughtfully organized, are provided for each topic.

www.macmillan.org.uk

Another excellent resource is Great Britain's Macmillan Cancer Support. Cancer treatment in Great Britain is very similar to that in the United States, and although the website uses slightly different terminology, it provides new perspectives.

www.aicr.org

The American Institute for Cancer Research is my favorite source of information related to cancer prevention.

Support Organizations

I encourage people to visit their nearest local cancer support organization. In Ithaca, NY, people often come to the Cancer Resource Center of the Finger Lakes (www.crcfl.net) when they are first diagnosed. They usually say something like, "I just found out that I have cancer, but I don't even know what questions to ask." We help them get their bearings by providing information and connecting them with others who have been through cancer treatment. Many communities have organizations like ours.

If your community doesn't have its own cancer support organization, many national cancer organizations have matching services to connect you with others with your specific disease.

www.acor.org
The Association of Cancer Online Resources offers online communities to connect with others with specific types of cancer.

www.sharethecare.org
www.lotsahelpinghands.com
Share the Care and Lotsa Helping Hands are excellent models of bringing friends together to support an individual needing assistance.

An increasing number of hospitals have nurse navigators whose job is to be a central point of contact for cancer patients. They can answer your questions or get you connected with the right person.

Index